Blackwell's Primary
Care Essentials:
Urology

Blackwell's Primary Care Essentials

Blackwell's Primary Care Essentials: Urology

Pamela Ellsworth, MD

Assistant Professor of Surgery/Urology
Dartmouth Medical School
Hanover, New Hampshire
Staff Urologist
Dartmouth Medical Center
Lebanon, New Hampshire

Stephen N. Rous, MD

Professor of Surgery/Urology
Dartmouth Medical School
Hanover, New Hampshire
Chief of Urology
Veterans Affairs Medical Center
White River Junction, Vermont

Series Editor

Daniel K. Onion, MD, MPH, FACP
Professor of Community and Family Medicine
Dartmouth Medical School
Director of Maine-Dartmouth Family Practice Residency Program
Augusta, Maine

Blackwell
Science

©2001 by Blackwell Science, Inc.

Editorial Offices:
Commerce Place, 350 Main Street, Malden, Massachusetts 02148, USA
Osney Mead, Oxford OX2 0EL, England
25 John Street, London WC1N 2BL, England
23 Ainslie Place, Edinburgh EH3 6AJ, Scotland
54 University Street, Carlton, Victoria 3053, Australia

Other Editorial Offices:
Blackwell Wissenschafts-Verlag GmbH, Kurfürstendamm 57, 10707 Berlin, Germany
Blackwell Science KK, MG Koden-macho Building, 7-10 Kodenmacho Nihombashi, Chuo-ku, Tokyo 104, Japan
Iowa State University Press, A Blackwell Science Company, 2121 S. State Avenue, Ames, Iowa 50014-8300, USA

Distributors:
The Americas
Blackwell Publishing
c/o AIDC
P.O. Box 20
50 Winter Sport Lane
Williston, VT 05495-0020
(Telephone orders: 800-216-2522; fax orders: 802-864-7626)

Canada
Login Brothers Book Company
324 Saulteaux Crescent
Winnipeg, Manitoba R3J 3T2
(Telephone orders: 204-837-2987)

Australia
Blackwell Science Pty, Ltd.
54 University Street
Carlton, Victoria 3053
(Telephone orders: 03-9347-0300; fax orders: 03-9349-3016)

Outside The Americas and Australia
Blackwell Science, Ltd.
c/o Marston Book Services, Ltd.
P.O. Box 269
Abingdon
Oxon OX14 4YN
England
(Telephone orders: 44-01235-465500; fax orders: 44-01235-465555)

Library of Congress Cataloging-in-Publication Data

Ellsworth, Pamela.
  Blackwell's primary care essentials.
Urology / Pamela Ellsworth, Stephen Rous.
    p. cm. — (Blackwell's primary care essentials series)
    ISBN 0-86542-585-X
    1. Urology—Handbooks, manuals, etc.
2. Genitourinary organs—Handbooks, manuals, etc. I. Rous, Stephen N. (Stephen Norman), 1931– . II. Blackwell Science.
III. Title. IV. Title: Urology. V. Series.
    [DNLM: 1. Urologic Diseases.
WJ 140 E47b 2001]
    RC872.9.E44 2001
    616.6—dc21

00-067463

Acquisitions: Nancy Anastasi Duffy
Development: William Deluise
Production: Andover Publishing Services
Manufacturing: Lisa Flanagan
Marketing Manager: Toni Fournier
Cover design by Leslie Haimes
Typeset by Graphicraft Limited, Hong Kong
Printed and bound by Edwards Brothers

Printed in the United States of America
01 02 03 04 5 4 3 2 1

The Blackwell Science logo is a trade mark of Blackwell Science Ltd., registered at the United Kingdom Trade Marks Registry

"The love of learning, the sequestered nooks, And all the sweet serenity of books"

—Henry Wadsworth Longfellow (Morituri Salutamus)

This book is gratefully dedicated to my parents in recognition of their inspiring guidance, most especially in my formative years. To my Father, who instilled in me a sense of the thrill, challenge, and satisfaction of lifelong learning. To my Mother, whose constant, enthusiastic and energetic example gave me an appreciation of the obligation to devote a piece of myself to the service of others.

P.E.

Contents

Section I   ADULT UROLOGY

Section II   PEDIATRIC UROLOGY

Preface

As a general surgery resident I became dismayed by the bulk of material that the "general surgeon" was expected to know. How, I thought, could one understand and know everything from the head to the toe? Urology, however, seemed so simple then—only the genitourinary tract. Now that could be mastered. It wasn't long into my urology residency that I realized there was a reason the leading textbook, *Campbell's Urology*, was in three volumes. However, at that time learning the material was not a chore. It was an interesting and exciting field, and I quickly realized that I had made the right choice.

Clearly, the field of urology cannot be adequately summarized in 200 pages or less. Rather, it is the intention of this book to provide an overview and discuss those subjects that are typically encountered in a general medical and urologic practice. It is my hope that the information contained in this book will answer the more common questions and that the references will provide as much in-depth information as may be desired by the readers. I hope that all who read this book will realize what an exciting and constantly evolving field urology is.

I would like to express my sincere thanks to my colleague, friend, and mentor, Stephen Rous, who epitomizes the role of mentor. Without his assistance and knowledge this book would not have been possible. In addition, I would like to thank Alicia Green, who spent many hours reviewing the text and preparing the tables. Her assistance was invaluable.

P. E.

Medical Abbreviations

AB	antibodies
ABG	arterial blood gas
abnl	abnormal, abnormality
abx	antibiotics
ACE	angiotensin converting enzyme
ACEI	ACE inhibitor
ADH	antidiuretic hormone
AFB	acid fast bacillus
AFP	alpha fetoprotein
ag	antigen
AGN	acute glomerular nephritis
aka	also known as
ANA	antinuclear antibody
AODM	adult onset diabetes mellitus
APR	abdominal perineal resection
ARDS	acute respiratory distress syndrome
ASCVD	arteriosclerotic heart disease
assoc	association/associated
asx	asymptomatic
BCG	Bacille Calmette Guerin
BM	bone marrow
BMT	bone marrow transplant
BPLND	bilateral pelvic lymph node dissection
BPH	benign prostatic hypertrophy
BOO	bladder outlet obstruction
btn	between
BUN	blood urea nitrogen
bx	biopsy
BXO	balanitis xerotica obliterans

Ca	calcium
CAD	coronary artery disease
cAMP	cyclic adenosinemonophosphate
CBC	complete blood count
CBI	continuous bladder irrigation
cc	cubic centimeter
CDC	Centers for Disease Control
CEA	carcinoembryonic antigen
CFU	colony forming unit
cGMP	cyclic guanosinemonophosphate
CHF	congestive heart failure
CIC	clean intermittent catheterization
CIS	carcinoma in situ
Cl	chloride
CMG	cystometrogram
cmplc	complications
c/o	complaining of
CO_2	carbon dioxide
Col	colonies
comb	combination
CP	cerebral palsy
CRH	corticotropin releasing hormone
crit	hematocrit
crs	course
c + s	culture and sensitivity
CT	computed tomography
CV	cardiovascular
CVA	cerebrovascular accident
cxray	chest x-ray
Cysto	cystoscopy
DAT	dementia, Alzheimer's type
d/c	discontinue
decr	decrease
DH	detrusor hyperreflexia
DI	detrusor instability
DM	diabetes mellitus
diffdx	differential diagnosis
DMSA	technetium-99m dimercaptosuccinic acid

DMSO	dimethyl sulfoxide
DRE	digital rectal examination
ds	double strength
dx	diagnosis or diagnostic
dz	disease
ED	erectile dysfunction
ELISA	enzyme linked immunosorbent assay
EMG	electromyelogram
ESR	erythrocyte sedimentation rate
ESWL	extracorporeal shock wave lithotripsy
f	female
FA	fluorescent antibody
FISH	fluorescent in-situ hybridization
FSH	follicle stimulating hormone
FTA	fluorescent treponemal antibody
f/u	follow up
GC	gonorrhea
GFR	glomerular filtration rate
GI	gastrointestinal
gm	gram
GN	glomerulonephritis
GU	genitourinary
h	hour
H^+	hydrogen
HA	headache
HCG	human chorionic gonadotropin
HCl	hydrochloride
HCO_3	bicarbonate
hct	hematocrit
H & E	hematoxylin and eosin
Hgb	hemoglobin
5-HIAA	5-hydroxyindolacetic acid
HIV	human immunodeficiency virus
HLA	human leukocyte antigens
h/o	history of

hpf	high power field
HPV	human papillomavirus
HSV	herpes simplex virus
HT	hypertension
5HT	5-hydroxytryptophan
HVA	homovanillic acid
hx	history
I or I_2	iodine
IC	intersititial cystitis
I & D	incision and drainage
IDDM	insulin dependent diabetes mellitus
IFA	immunofluorescent antibody
IgA	immunoglobulin A
IgE	immunoglobulin E
IgG	immunoglobulin G
IgM	immunoglobulin M
im	intramuscular
incl	include, including, included
INH	isoniazid
IU	international units
iv	intravenous
IVP	intravenous pyelogram
K	potassium
kg	kilogram
KOH	potassium hydroxide
KUB	abdominal x-ray—"kidneys, ureter, bladder"
L	liter or left
lab(s)	laboratory tests
lat	lateral
LDH	lactate dehydrogenase
LFT	liver function test
LH	luteinizing hormone
LHRH	LH releasing hormone
LMW	low molecular weight
LUTS	lower urinary tract symptoms
lytes	electrolytes

m	male
Mag 3	technetium-99m mercaptoacetyl triglycerine
MAO	monoamine oxidase
MCDK	multicystic dysplastic kidney
med(s)	medication(s)
MEN	multiple endocrine neoplasias
mets	metastases
mEq	milliequivalent
mg	milligram
MG	magnesium
MI	myocardial infarction
mL	milliliter
mo	month
MRI	magnetic resonance imaging
MS	multiple sclerosis
MSH	melanocyte stimulating hormone
Mtx	methotrexate
μgm	microgram

Na	sodium
NCI	National Cancer Institute
Nd:Yag	neodymium–yttrium aluminum garnet
NH_3	ammonia
NIH	National Institutes of Health
nl	normal
nL	nanoliter
NSAID	nonsteroidal anti-inflammatory drug
N/V	nausea, vomiting

PA	posteroanterior
PABA	paraminobenzoic acid
PCR	polymerase chain reaction
Pg	prostaglandin
Pheo	pheochromocytoma
Phos	phosphorous
Polys	polymorphonuclear cells
pos	positive
PPD	tuberculin skin test
PSA	prostate specific antigen

pt(s)	patient(s)
PTH	parathyroid hormone
PV sling	pubovaginal sling
PVR	post void residual
RBC	red blood cell
RCC	renal cell carcinoma
RIA	radioimmunoassay
r/o	rule out
RPLND	retroperitoneal lymph node dissection
RPR	rapid plasma reagin (test for syphilis)
RRPX	radical retropubic prostatectomy
RTA	renal tubular acidosis
rx	treatment/treated/therapy
si	signs
sl	sublingual
s/p	status post
specif	specificity
SS	sickle cell disease
Staph	staphylococcus
STD	sexually transmitted disease
STS	serologic test for syphilis
SUI	stress urinary incontinence
sx	symptoms
sxic	symptomatic
tab	tablet
TAH	total abdominal hysterectomy
TB	tuberculosis
TBI	total body irradiation
TCC	transitional cell carcinoma
Tm	trimethoprim
Tm/S	trimethoprim/sulfa
TNF	tumor necrosis factor
Tng	nitroglycerine
TNM	tumor, nodes, mets
TPN	total parenteral nutrition
TRUS	transrectal ultrasound
tsp	teaspoon

TUR	transurethral resection
TURBT	transurethral resection bladder tumor
TURP	transurethral resection of the prostate
U	units
UA	urinalysis
UDT	undescended testis
UPJ	ureteropelvic junction
UPJO	UPJ obstruction
UPP	urethral pressure profile
US	ultrasound
UTI	urinary tract infection
UVJ	ureterovesical junction
VCUG	voiding cystourethrogram
VDRL	Venereal Disease Research Laboratory (serologic test for syphilis)
VIP	vasoactive intestinal peptide
VLPP	Valsalva leak point pressure
VMA	vanillylmandelic acid
vol	volume
VUR	vesicoureteral reflux
VURD	valve unilateral reflux and dysplasia
w/up	work up
WBC	white blood cells
wk	week
XGP	xanthogranulomatous pyelonephritis
XRT	radiation therapy
yr	year
More than	>
Much more than	>>
Less than	<
Much less than	<<

Journal Abbreviations

A J Roentgenol	American Journal of Roentgenology
ACS	American Cancer Society
Acta Pediatr Scan	Acta Paediatrica Scandinavica
Acta Trop	Acta Tropica
Acta Urol Belg	Acta Urologica Belgica
Adv Int Med	Advances in Internal Medicine
Adv Ped	Advances in Pediatrics
Adv Urol	Advances in Urology
AJR	American Journal of Radiology
Am J Anat	American Journal of Anatomy
Am J Clin Nutr	American Journal of Clinical Nutrition
Am J Clin Path	American Journal of Clinical Pathology
Am J Dis Child	American Journal of Diseases of Childhood
Am J Hum Genet	American Journal of Human Genetics
Am J Kidney	American Journal of Kidney
Am J Kidney Dis	American Journal of Kidney Disease
Am J Med	American Journal of Medicine
Am J Nephrol	American Journal of Nephrology
Am J Obstet Gynecol	American Journal of Obstetrics and Gynecology
Am J Pathol	American Journal of Pathology
Am J Public Health	American Journal of Public Health
Am J Radiol	American Journal of Radiology
Am J Surg Path	American Journal of Surgical Pathology
Am J Trop Med Hyg	American Journal of Tropical Medicine and Hygiene

Am Rev Resp Dis	American Review of Respiratory Disease
Am Surg	American Surgeon
Ann Emerg Med	Annals of Emergency Medicine
Ann IM	Annals of Internal Medicine
Ann Paeditr Fenn	Annals Paediatriae Fenniae
Ann Soc Belg Med Trop	Annales de Societe Belge de Medicine Tropicale
Ann Surg	Annals of Surgery
Antimicrob Agents Chemother	Antimicrobial Agents and Chemotherapy
Antiviral Res	Antiviral Research
Arch Androl	Archives of Andrology
Arch Derm	Archives of Dermatology
Arch Dis Child	Archives of Diseases of Childhood
Arch IM	Archives of Internal Medicine
Arch Klin Chir	Archiv der Klinischen Chirurgie
Arch Pathol	Archives of Pathology
Arch Pathol Lab Med	Archives of Pathology and Laboratory Medicine
AUA Update	American Urological Association Update Series
Aud Dig	Audio Digest
Aust NZ J Surg	Australia New Zealand Journal of Surgery
Aust NZ Obstet Gynecol	Australia New Zealand Obstetrics and Gynecology
Behav Res Ther	Behaviour Research and Therapy
Biochem Biophys Res Commun	Biochemical & Biophysical Research Communications
BMJ	British Medical Journal
Br J Hosp Med	British Journal of Hospital Medicine
BJU	British Journal of Urology
Br J Radiol	British Journal of Radiology
Br J Surg	British Journal of Surgery
Br J Vener Dis	British Journal of Venereal Disease
Bull Rheum Dis	Bulletin of Rheumatic Disease
Bull WHO	Bulletin of the World Health Organization

Can J Surg	Canadian Journal of Surgery
Can Med Assoc J	Canadian Medical Association Journal
Cancer Res	Cancer Research
Clin Infect Dis	Clinical Infectious Disease
Clin Obstet Gynecol	Clinical Obstetrics and Gynecology
Clin Oncol	Clinical Oncology
Clin Ped	Clinical Pediatrics
Clin Radiol	Clinical Radiology
Curr Opin Rheum	Current Opinions in Rheumatology
Curr Opin Urol	Current Opinions in Urology
Derm	Dermatology
Derm Clin	Dermatology Clinics
Derm Surg	Dermatologic Surgery
Diagn Cytopathol	Diagnostic Cytopathology
Dialogues Pediatr Urol	Dialogues in Pediatric Urology
Emerg Med Clin North Am	Emergency Medicine Clinics of North America
Endocrin	Endocrinology
Epidem	Epidemiology
Epidemiol Rev	Epidemiologic Review
Eur J Pediatr	European Journal of Pediatrics
Eur J Radiol	European Journal of Radiology
Eur Urol	European Urology
Fertil Steril	Fertility and Sterility
Fogarty Int Center Proc	Fogarty International Center Proceedings
Fortschr Roentgenstr	Fortschritte auf dem Gebiete der Roentgenstrahlen
GE	Gastroenterology
Gen Clin Pathol	General Clinical Pathology
Genes Chromosom Cancer	Genes, Chromosomes and Cancer
Genitourin Med	Genitourinary Medicine
Gerontol Clin	Gerontology Clinics

Hematol Oncol Clin North Am	Hematology & Oncology Clinics of North America
Histochem J	Histochemical Journal
Histopath	Histopathology
Hum Genet	Human Genetics
Hum Pathol	Human Pathology
Hum Reprod	Human Reproduction
Infect Dis Clin North Am	Infectious Disease Clinics of North America
Infect Urol	Infections in Urology
Int J Cancer	International Journal of Cancer
Int J Derm	International Journal of Dermatology
Int J Impot Res	International Journal of Impotence Research
Int J Urol	International Journal of Urology
Int Surg	International Surgery
Int Urol Nephrol	International Urology and Nephrology
Johns Hopkins Med J	Johns Hopkins Medical Journal
Jama	Journal of the American Medical Association
J Am Acad Derm	Journal of the American Academy of Dermatology
J Androl	Journal of Andrology
J Antimicrob Chemo	Journal of Antimicrobial Chemotherapy
J Bone Joint Surg	Journal of Bone and Joint Surgery
J Clin Endocrinol Metab	Journal of Clinical Endocrinology & Metabolism
J Clin Oncol	Journal of Clinical Oncology
J Clin Pathol	Journal of Clinical Pathology
J Computed Assisted Tomography	Journal of Computed Assisted Tomography
J Computed Tomography	Journal of Computed Tomography
J Contin Ed Urol	Journal of Continuing Education In Urology

J Derm Surg Onc	Journal of Dermatologic Surgery and Oncology
J d'Urologie	Journal d'Urologie
J Endourol	Journal of Endourology
J Infect Dis	Journal of Infectious Disease
J Invest Derm	Journal of Investigative Dermatology
J Leukoc Biol	Journal of Leukocyte Biology
J Med Genet	Journal of Medical Genetics
J Musculoskel Pain	Journal of Musculoskeletal Pain
J NCI	Journal of the National Cancer Institute
J Natl Med Assoc	Journal of the National Medical Association
J Neurosurg	Journal of Neurosurgery
J Nucl Med	Journal of Nuclear Medicine
J Ocul Pharmacol	Journal of Ocular Pharmacology
J Pathol	Journal of Pathology
J Ped	Journal of Pediatrics
J Pediatr Surg	Journal of Pediatric Surgery
J Reprod Med	Journal of Reproductive Medicine
J Trauma	Journal of Trauma
J Urol	Journal of Urology
Kidney Int	Kidney International
Klin Paediatr	Klinische Paediatrie
Mayo Clin Proc	Mayo Clinic Proceedings
Med	Medicine
Med Grand Rounds	Medical Grand Rounds
Med Let	Medical Letter
Miner Electrol Metab	Mineral & Electrolyte Metabolism
Mmwr	CDC Morbidity and Mortality Weekly Review
Mod Concepts Cardiovasc Dis	Modern Concepts in Cardiovascular Disease
Mod Pathol	Modern Pathology
Mol Cell Biol	Molecular Cell Biology
Mol Cell Prob	Molecular and Cellular Probes

Natur genet	Nature Genetics
NCI	National Cancer Institutes
Nejm	New England Journal of Medicine
Nephrol Dial Transplant	Nephrology, Dialysis, Transplantation
Neurourol Urodynam	Neurourology and Urodynamics
NY State Med J	New York State Medical Journal
Obstet Gynecol	Obstetrics and Gynecology
Ped Infect Dis J	Pediatric Infectious Disease Journal
Ped Nephrol	Pediatric Nephrology
Pediatr Clin North Am	Pediatric Clinics of North America
Pediatr Kidney Dis	Pediatric Kidney Diseases
Pediatr Med Clin	Pediatric Medical Clinics
Pediatr Radiol	Pediatric Radiology
Pediatr Surg Int	Pediatric Surgery International
Pediatr Urol	Pediatric Urology
Peds	Pediatrics
Postgrad Med	Postgraduate Medicine
Prenat Diagn	Prenatal Diagnosis
Proc Am Ass Cancer Res	Proceedings of the American Association of Cancer Research
Proc Eur Dial Transplant Assoc	Proceedings of the European Dialysis & Transplant Association
Proc Natl Acad Sci	Proceedings of the National Academy of Science
Proc R Soc Med	Proceedings of the Royal Society of Medicine
Rad Med	Radiation Medicine
Radiol Clin North Am	Radiology Clinics of North America
Rehab Lit	Rehabilitation Literature
Rev Infect Dis	Review in Infectious Disease
S Afr Med	South African Medicine
Scan J Infect Dis	Scandinavian Journal of Infectious Disease
Scan J Urol	Scandinavian Journal of Urology

Scan J Urol Nephrol	Scandinavian Journal of Urology and Nephrology
Semin Oncol	Seminars in Oncology
Semin Roentgenol	Seminars in Roentgenology
Semin Urol Oncol	Seminars in Urologic Oncology
Sex Transm Dis	Sexually Transmitted Disease
Sex Transm Infect	Sexually Transmitted Infections
Southern Med J	Southern Medical Journal
Surg Gynecol Obstet	Surgery, Gynecology and Obstetrics
Tech Urol	Techniques in Urology
Tex Med	Texas Medicine
Tex Rep Biol Med	Texas Reports on Biology and Medicine
Tokai J Exp Clin Med	Tokai Journal of Experimental & Clinical Medicine
Trans R Soc Trop Med Hyg	Transactions of Royal Society of Tropical Medicine & Hygiene
Urol Clin North Am	Urologic Clinics of North America
Urol Int	Urology International
Urol Radiol	Urologic Radiology
Virchows Arch	Virchows Archiv
Virchows Arch Path Anat	Virchows Archiv in Pathologie & Anatomie
World J Urol	World Journal of Urology

Notice

The indications and dosages of all drugs in this book have been recommended in the medical literature and conform to the practices of the general community. The medications described do not necessarily have specific approval by the Food and Drug Administration for use in the diseases and dosages for which they are recommended. The package insert for each drug should be consulted for use and dosage as approved by the FDA. Because standards for usage change, it is advisable to keep abreast of revised recommendations, particularly those concerning new drugs.

Section I

ADULT UROLOGY

1 Diseases of the Adrenal

1.1 CUSHING'S SYNDROME

Nejm 1995;332:791; Nejm 1994;331:629 (NIH-children)

Cause: (Nejm 1991;325:899): Chromophobe or basophilic micro- or macroadenoma of pituitary. Ectopic ACTH production by oat cell or other (ovary, pancreas, carcinoid) cancer; at least some of this type may be corticotropin hormone-releasing factor producers causing ACTH release indirectly through pituitary (Nejm 1971;285:419); occasionally ACTH-producing carcinoid tumors, especially of lung (Ann IM 1992;117:209). Adrenal: bilateral nodular hyperplasia or unilateral adenoma (15%) or carcinoma (<1% adults, 4% children with Cushing's in NIH study)

Pathophys: Glucocorticoids cause connective tissue dissolution; have anti-vitamin D effect; cause proteolysis of muscle, lymphocyte/monocyte inhibition (Nejm 1975;292:236), increased acid/pepsin secretion, increased gluconeogenesis, decreased glucose uptake. Aldosterone and androgens elevated too when ACTH is the mechanism

Sx: Muscle weakness, obesity/weight gain; growth retardation in children; easy bruising

Si: Muscle weakness, ecchymoses, moon face, buffalo hump, abdominal striae, truncal fat, osteoporosis and fractures, increased number and severity of infections, peptic ulcers, DM, nonketotic insulin-resistant, psychoses, virilization, HT (47% in children), edema

Crs: Excellent prognosis unless cancer or ectopic ACTH (usually cancer) (Nejm 1971;285:243)

Lab:

Chem: Serum cortisol, normal level 10–25 µgm% (= 280–700 nM/L) in am, dropping to <7 µgm% in pm; after 1 mg dexamethasone at 11 pm, 8 am cortisol is <5 in normal; if >10, r/o Cushing's (100% sens, 90% specif [Ann IM 1990;112:738]); false pos with phenytoin (Dilantin) (Aud Dig 1983;30:18). If indeterminate, 0.5 mg dexamethasone q6 h × 48 h and measure cortisol; or get 24-h urinary free cortisol (6% false neg, fewer false pos [Aud Dig 1983;30:18]) and/or 24-h urine cortisol × 3 ≥100 µgm/24 h

If above tests abnl, high-dose tests are done to differentiate cause (baseline 8 am cortisol, 8 mg dexamethasone at 11 pm, then 8 am cortisol). Pituitary Cushing's pts, unlike adrenal tumors or ectopic ACTH production types, suppress value to <50% of baseline value (92% sens, 100% specif [Ann IM 1986;104:180], 68% sens in children (Nejm 1994;330:1295 for various test sens and specif)

CRH Test: ACTH and cortisol increased after CRH given if pituitary tumor, not if ectopic ACTH or adrenal tumor (Ann IM 1985;102:344); 80% sens in children

Petrosal venous sampling for ACTH levels, simultaneous bilaterally reliably lateralize pituitary tumor (Nejm 1985;312:100)

Xray: (Ann IM 1988;109:547,613)

CT: 60% false-neg rate due to small adenomas

MRI with gadolinium enhancement: 71% sens (52% sens in children), 87% specif; but 10% of normal adult population will have a lesion (Ann IM 1994;120:817)

Rx: 1st: Surgical transsphenoidal microadenomectomy, 90% successful (Nejm 1984;310:889) vs 76% (Ann IM 1988;109:487); bilateral adrenalectomy. 2nd: Irradiation of pituitary, 83% successful in pts for whom surgery failed (Nejm 1997;336:172). 3rd: Aminoglutethimide, mitotane, metyrapone, trilostane (Med Let 1985;27:87); bromocriptine; ketoconazole for antisteroid synthesis effect (Nejm 1987;317:812)

1.2 CONN'S SYNDROME

Nejm 1994;331:250

Cause: Bilateral adrenal hyperplasia or unilateral adrenal adenoma-secreting aldosterone

Epidem: 1% of all hypertensive pts? (Ann IM 1970;72:9)

Pathophys: Increased aldosterone production causes Na^+ retention and K^+ loss, leading to hypervolemia of 2–3 L; HT; H^+ loss, causing metabolic alkalosis. Is there an anterior pituitary "aldosterone simulating factor?" (Nejm 1984;311:120)

Sx: Fatigue, weakness, tetany

Si: HT; Trousseau's si, due to alkalosis; little edema, unlike secondary causes of increased aldosterone; proximal myopathy

Cmplc: r/o Liddle's syndrome, an aldosterone-like effect caused by autosomal dominantly inherited renal tubular defect (Nejm 1994;330:178). Bartter's syndrome and licorice ingestion (Nejm 1991;325:1223), both of which cause a normotensive hyperaldosteronism by peripheral angiotensin resistance and/or prostaglandin induction (Ann IM 1977;281:369; Nejm 1973;289:1022); rx with NSAIDs, especially indomethacin (Ann IM 1977;87:281). Secondary causes of hyperaldosteronism. Rare unilateral adenoma or cancer of adrenal (Ann IM 1984;101:316)

Lab:

Chem: Aldosterone levels elevated; elevated Na^+; K^+ <3.7 mEq/L suspicious; HCO_3 elevated; renin levels low, but elevated in secondary types of hyperaldosteronism. Adrenal vein sampling for lateralized aldosterone and cortisol levels

Saline Infusion Test: 2 L NaCl iv over 4 h decreases serum aldosterone to <10 ng% in normals (Ann IM 1984;100:300)

Captopril Test: 25 mg po × 1 decreases serum aldosterone levels to <50% at 2 h in normals (Ann IM 1984;100:300) but not if Conn's present

Xray: CT very good to dx operable adenoma vs inoperable bilateral hyperplasia (Nejm 1980;303:1503)

Rx: Spironolactone 100 mg qid; cyproheptadine? (Nejm 1981;305:181). Surgical adrenalectomy when unilateral lesion, though BP cured by this in only 35% (Ann IM 1995;122:877)

1.3 ADDISON'S DISEASE (PRIMARY ADRENAL INSUFFICIENCY)

Nejm 1996;335:1206

Cause: Idiopathic; autoimmune suppressor T-cell defect (Nejm 1979;300:164); metastatic cancer; infection, especially TB, and meningococcemia with Friderichsen–Waterhouse syndrome; stress in pt chronically suppressed with steroids, possibly even inhaled beclomethasone (Nejm 1978;299:1387); HIV in AIDS pts (Ann IM 1997;127:1103)

Epidem: Peak incidence age 20–40. Associated with HLA-B8 and DR 3/4, and thereby with pernicious anemia, myasthenia gravis, islet cell antibody IDDM, myxedema, vitiligo, alopecia, primary gonadal failure

Pathophys: 80% of gland must be destroyed to get sx. ACTH and MSH similar, hence increased pigmentation; both mineralocorticoid and glucocorticoid deficiencies create si/sx

Sx: Loss of sense of well-being; increased pigmentation, especially of scars, creases, buccal mucosa; N/V, diarrhea, salt craving, weight loss; rarely galactorrhea (Nejm 1972;287:1326)

Si: Hypotension, postural first and later even supine; cachexia; hyperpigmentation, vitiligo, longitudinal nail pigment streaks (Nejm 1969;281:1056); diminished axillary and pubic hair

Crs: 40% develop other glandular failure (especially thyroid and gonadal)

Cmplc: r/o hyporeninemic hypoaldosteronism with hyperkalemia and metabolic acidosis due to depressed prostaglandin synthesis (Nejm 1986;314:1015,1041) seen in AODM and primary renal disease. Adrenoleukodystrophy in boys, a sex-linked abnormality of fatty acid metabolism (Nejm 1990;322:13). Autoimmune polyendocrinopathy candidiasis/ectodermal dystrophy (Nejm 1990;322:1829); 80% are hypoparathyroid, 70% are hypoadrenal, 60% of women are hypogonadal compared to 15% of men; by age 20, 100% have had significant candidal infections

Lab:

Chem: Na low, HCO_3 low, K elevated, ACTH elevated. 8 am cortisol <3 μgm is diagnostic; <15 μgm% when under stress; if >20 μgm%, dx unlikely (D. Spratt 1/94)

Cosyntropin screening test of adrenal reserve: Get fasting blood cortisol, give 250 μgm cosyntropin (ACTH analog) iv and draw repeat cortisol 30 min later (or im and 60 min later); a normal increases >6 μgm% to >20 μgm% if adequate adrenal reserve (Nejm 1976;295:30)

Hem: CBC may show eosinophilia

Rx: Glucocorticoids like cortisol 25–30 mg po qd in am to mimic early am peaks; steroid equivalents in order of diminishing mineralocorticoid component: hydrocortisone 20 mg, prednisone 5 mg, methylprednisolone 4 mg, dexamethasone 0.75 mg. Mineralocorticoid, eg, fludrocortisone (Fluorinef) 100–300 μgm qd; adjust dose by renin level, which should be normal if adequate replacement; can cause significant supine HT over years (Nejm 1979;301:68). Androgens can help reestablish sense of well-being, especially in females, but use cautiously

In steroid-induced adrenal suppression (Nejm 1997;337:1285), slow tapering of steroids (Nejm 1976;295:30) to allow recovery of pituitary–adrenal axis, decrease to physiologic level of 20 mg hydrocortisone or other steroid equivalent qam, then taper q4 wk to 10 mg qd by 2.5-mg increments; when 8 am plasma cortisol before pills is >10 μgm%, stop and expect baseline adrenal function to be ok; still must supplement with 50 mg hydrocortisone or equivalent bid for minor and 100 mg tid for major illnesses. When cosyntropin test (see under "Lab") is normal, no longer need such supplementation (Nejm 1976;295:30)

1.4 PHEOCHROMOCYTOMA (PHEO)

Cause: Neoplasm of adrenal gland or extra-adrenal autonomic ganglia

Epidem: Causative factor in <1% of the hypertensive population. 10% of pheos found in normotensive individuals. 95% are isolated anomalies, 5% are autosomal dominant, possible chromosome 19 (Nejm 1996;335:945, Jama 1995;274:1149). Familial pheos may be divided into different types of genetic abnormalities. MEN 2 syndrome characterized by pheo, medullary carcinoma of the thyroid, and parathyroid adenoma. MEN 3 characterized by pheo, medullary carcinoma of the thyroid, mucosal neuromas, thickened corneal nerves, alimentary tract, ganglioneuromatosis, and frequently marfanoid habitus (Cancer Surv 1990;9:703); the neuroectodermal dysplasias including von Recklinhausen's disease (neurofibromatosis), tuberous sclerosis (see angiomyolipoma), Sturge–Weber syndrome, and von Hippel–Lindau disease. In contrast to adults, children demonstrate a higher incidence of familial pheo (10%) and bilateral disease (24%) (Campbell's Urology 1998;7(2):2915–2972). Rule of 10s applies: 10% familial, 10% extra-adrenal, 10% bilateral, 10% malignant for adults

Pathophys: Clinical manifestations of pheo are related to physiologic effects of amines that it produces. Lesions typically produce epinephrine and norepinephrine, but other unusual products include dopamine, dopa, and peptides produced by the amine precursor and decarboxylation (APUD) cells (Hum Pathol 1974;51:409; Robertson, D: The adrenal medulla and adreno-medullary hoemones. In Scott HW (ed): Surgery of the Adrenal Glands. Philadelphia: JB Lippincott, 1990)

Sx: Headache, excessive sweating, palpitations, anxiety or nervousness, chest or abdominal discomfort, N/V, weight loss, warmth, dyspnea, visual disturbances, dizziness, constipation, shock, paresthesia or pain in arm, seizure

Si: HT sustained, paroxysmal, or sustained with superimposed paroxysmal (Surgery 1982;91:367), orthostatic systolic blood pressure drop, hyperhidrosis, tachycardia, facial and upper body pallor, hypertensive retinopathy, anxiousness, dilated pupils, tremor, underweight, Raynaud's phenomenon, palpable mass, mass effects

Crs: May be underlying causative agent in pts presenting with diseases that may result from excess catecholamine production, including CVAs, encephalopathy, retinopathy, CHF, cardiomyopathy, dissecting aneurysm, ARDS, shock, renal failure, azotemia, ischemic enterocolitis, megacolon (Campbell's Urology 1998;7(3):2915–2972)

Cmplc: Includes catecholamine-induced cardiomyopathy, CVA, MI, renovascular disease, renal insufficiency, ischemic enterocolitis

DiffDx: Variety of disorders may cause similar si/sx incl anxiety, hyperthyroidism, menopause, DM, autonomic dysreflexia, toxemia of pregnancy, adrenocortical carcinoma, acute infectious disease, neurofibromatosis, migraine, intracranial lesion, cerebrovascular disease, paroxysmal tacchycardia (Manger W, Gifford RW Jr: Pheochromocytoma. In Laragh JH, Brenner BM, eds: Hypertension: Pathophysiology, Diagnosis and Management. New York, Raven, 1990)

Lab: Elevated levels of catecholamines (norepinephrine, dopamine, and epinephrine) in blood or urine and elevated urinary metanephrines in 95–99% of affected individuals (Campbell's Urology 1998;7(3):2915–2972)

Chem: Plasma catechols >2000 pgm/cc, supine 30 min after needle placed, best test, 5–10% false neg, no false pos. Clonidine-suppression test if plasma catechols 1000–2000: 0.3 mg po with plasma norepinephrine level before and at 3 h; all normals suppress to <300 pg/cc (Nejm 1991;305:623). Plasma metanephrines as good or better than (Ann IM 1995;123:101,150)

24-h urine metanephrines, 5% false-pos rate, 2% false-neg rate, 50% pos predictive value, or metanephrine/creatinine ratio >0.354 is even better (Ann IM 1996;125:300); VMA, 20–60% false-neg rate; catechols, especially free norepinephrines, 80–100% sens, 98% specif (Nejm 1988;319:136)

Xray: CT scan is accurate in more than 90% of cases (Am J Radiol 1980;135:477). MRI is as accurate as a CT scan—characteristic bright "light bulb" appearance of T2-weighted study (Radiology 1986;158:81)—and also gives information on vasculature. Metaiodobenzylguanidine (MIBG) scan useful to identify residual, multiple, and extra adrenal lesions: 78.4% sens with primary sporadic tumors, 92.4% in malignant tumors, 94.3% in familial tumors (Southern Med J 1991;84:1221; J Nucl Med 1985;26:576)

Rx: Surgical removal after adequate preoperative preparation. Phenoxybenzamine hydrochloride (dibenzyline), 20–30 mg initially, increasing by 10–20 mg/d until blood pressure is stable and there is mild postural hypotension. Usually requires daily dose of 40–100 mg. Propranolol used when cardiac arrythmias are prominent, but may only be used when effective alpha-blockade is established. Dosage of 20–40 mg po tid to qid. Alpha-methylparatyrosine (metyrosine) decreases catecholamine synthesis. It is used in patients with cardiomyopathy and resistance to alpha-blockers. Dose is 0.5–1.0 g po 3–4 times per day. Side effects include crystalluria, sedation, diarrhea, anxiety, and psychiatric disturbance. All patients should be adequately hydrated. Anesthetic considerations: Induction with iv agent such as thiopental, followed by isoflurane as inhalation agent. Avoid propofol, ketamine, halothane, droperidol, morphine, and select skeletal muscle relaxants. Treat intraoperative HT with phentolamine or sodium nitroprusside. Surgical rx is laparoscopic adrenalectomy or via transabdominal approach (Chevron or thoracoabdominal incision). For metastatic lesions, combination chemotherapy is employed (Ann IM 1988;109:267)

2 Diseases of the Kidney and Ureter

2.1 ACUTE PYELONEPHRITIS

Ann IM 1989;111:906

Cause: Gram-negative rods in 95% of cases. Most commonly *E. coli* (particularly uropathic strains) (Nejm 1985;313:44). Other responsible organisms include *Klebsiella*, *Proteus*, *Enterobacter*, *Pseudomonas*, *Serratia*, *Citrobacter*, *Enterococcus faecalis*, *Staphylococcus aureus*. May be via ascending or hematogenous route

Epidem: Females > males. Increased incidence in pts with urologic instrumentation (Nejm 1974;291:215), congenital urinary tract anomalies, papillary necrosis, Sickle cell disease, DM, chronic indwelling catheters

Pathophys: Increased bacterial resistance appears to be necessary to overcome host resistance factors. Most cases caused by retrograde ascent of bacteria from bladder through ureter to renal pelvis and renal parenchyma. VUR, special bacterial adhesions (p. pili), and any process that interferes with normal ureteral peristalsis (obstruction, bacterial endotoxins) may facilitate bacterial ascent. Elevated renal pelvic pressure due to obstruction or reflux enhances ascent into the collecting tubules. May be a predisposition to infections of renal medulla due to increased osmotic pressure which causes white cell inhibition, decreased blood flow, and NH_3 inhibition of C′4 complement

Sx: Fever, flank pain, frequency, urgency, dysuria, hematuria, nausea

Si: CVA punch tenderness

Crs: Fever and flank pain persist for several days after initiation of abx. If sx persist for longer than 72 h, further evaluation for an abscess, urinary tract anomaly, and/or obstruction is indicated. 10–30% of pts with acute pyelonephritis have a relapse after 14-d course of rx. In these pts, additional 2-wk course is indicated. Rarely, pts require 6 wk of abx (Infect Dis Clin North Am 1987;1:773; Antimicrob Agents Chemother 1984;25:626)

Cmplc: Renal scarring, renal failure, HT, chronic pyelonephritis, emphysematous pyelonephritis. Children are at increased risk for scarring with pyelonephritis

DiffDx: Cystitis, intercourse-induced increased bacteriuria (Nejm 1978;298:321), renal abscess, acute interstitial nephritis (Ann IM 1980;93:735), and cystitis with VUR by doing VCUG

Perinephric abscess—located within Gerota's fascia—may be cmplc of pyelonephritis or occur secondary to hematogenous spread. Two factors differentiate acute pyelonephritis from perinephric abscess: (1) pts with uncomplicated pyelonephritis often have sx <5 d prior to hospitalization, whereas those with perinephric abscess have sx longer; and (2) pts with pyelonephritis often afebrile within 4 d of abx whereas those with perinephric abscess tend to be febrile for longer periods despite abx (Medicine 1974;53:441). Renal US or CT will help localize the perinephric abscess (Urol Clin North Am 1982;9:219). Rx consists of abx and drainage, either via an open approach or percutaneous drainage (Medicine 1988;67:118)

Lab: UA (microscopic), c + s from a midstream urine or catheterized urine sample. Gram stain of unspun urine shows ≥1 bacterium/oil immersion field. In a sx pt, urine c + s demonstrating >10^2 CFU/mL is significant. Ab-coated bacteria tests are typically pos in pts with pyelonephritis. These may be neg early in disease and when humoral immune system is incompletely developed (as in an infant), and may also be pos in cystitis (Peds 1979;63:467; Acta Peadiatr Scan 1978;67:275)

Xray: IVP: 20% demonstrate generalized or focal renal enlargement (Radiology 1976;118:65). Obstruction of renal tubules from parenchymal edema and vasoconstriction may impair contrast excretion and lead to diminished nephrogram and delayed visualization of calyces (Radiology 1976;118:65). Dilation of ureter and renal pelvis in absence of obstruction may also be noted (Clin Radiol 1978;30:59; Radiology 1976;118:65). CT scan not routinely indicated unless sx do not improve. May demonstrate abscess formation

Rx: In an uncomplicated infection, outpatient rx may be considered including oral fluoroquinolones or Tm/S pending sensitivities for 14 days. In complicated infections, pt should be admitted and treated with hydration and iv abx, ampicillin plus aminoglycoside pending sensitivities for 14–21 d. Repeat urine cultures 5–7 d after start of therapy and 4–6 wk posttreatment (Campbell's Urology 1998;7(2):533–614)

2.2 EMPHYSEMATOUS PYELONEPHRITIS

Arch IM 2000;160(6):797.

Cause: Acute necrotizing parenchymal and perirenal infection by gas-forming organisms. *E. coli* is most frequently identified organism. *Klebsiella* and *Proteus* less common

Epidem: Usually occurs in diabetic pts. May also occur in pts with urinary tract obstruction assoc with calculi or papillary necrosis and significant renal impairment. Adults > children; females > males

Pathophys: Exact pathogenesis unknown. High glucose levels (in DM) in tissues may provide substrate for CO_2 production from glucose fermentation (Am J Med 1968;44:134). Also postulated that impaired host response, caused by local factors such as obstruction and medical disease, allows bacteria to use necrotic tissue to generate gas

Sx: Fever, vomiting, flank pain, urgency, frequency, dysuria

Si: CVA punch tenderness

Crs: Appears to be cmplc of severe pyelonephritis. 43% mortality rate (J Contin Ed Urol 1979;18:9)

Cmplc: May require nephrectomy. Assoc with increased mortality

DiffDx: Acute pyelonephritis—may have air in collecting system with acute pyelonephritis and a gas-producing bacteria; renal abscess

Lab: UA, c + s; CBC, lytes, BUN, creatinine, glucose

Xray: KUB: Intraparenchymal gas, may appear as mottled gas shadows over kidney or as crescentic collection of gas over upper pole of kidney. Gas may be identified in perinephric space or retroperitoneum. IVP not helpful, as affected kidney is poorly functioning. US may show strong focal echoes that suggest intraparenchymal gas (Am J Radiol 1979;132:656; Am J Radiol

1979;132:395). CT scan may be helpful in localizing gas and demonstrating extent of infection (Arch IM 2000;160(6):797)

Rx: Fluid resuscitation, abx, relief of obstruction if present. If no improvement, surgical drainage or nephrectomy indicated (Am J Med 1968;44:134). In select cases percutaneous drainage and abx can be used successfully (Clin Radiol 1988;39:622)

2.3 RENAL ABSCESS

Cause: Prior to abx era, 80% of renal abscesses were attributed to hematogenous seeding by *Staphylococcus* (Surg Gynecol Obstet 1930;51:654). Over past two decades, gram-negative organisms are the cause of the majority of adult abscesses, and access the kidney via retrograde ascent

Epidem: 2/3 of gram-negative abscesses in adults are assoc with renal calculi or damaged kidneys (J Urol 1967;98:296). Association btn VUR and renal abscess is rarely noted (J Urol 1973;109:1029)

Pathophys: Complicated UTI assoc with stasis, calculi, malignancy, neurogenic bladder, and DM appear to predispose to abscess formation (Urol 1980;16:333). Most commonly related to ascending infection assoc with tubular obstruction from prior infections or calculi

Sx: Fever, chills, malaise, urgency, frequency, dysuria

Si: Abdominal or flank pain and weight loss

Crs: Small lesions may resolve spontaneously with IV abx; larger lesions often require drainage

Cmplc: Sepsis, loss of renal function

DiffDx: Pyelonephritis, renal tumor

Lab: CBC demonstrates marked leukocytosis; blood cultures usually positive. UA, c + s often pos, but may be neg in setting of hematogenous spread

Xray: Xray findings depend on nature and duration of infection. CT scan is radiologic test of choice. Initially CT scan may show renal enlargement and focal, rounded areas of decreased attenuation. After several days there may be a thick fibrotic wall around the abscess. Chronic abscess reveals obliteration of tissue planes, thickening of Gerota's fascia, and low-attenuation parenchymal mass surrounded by an inflammatory wall of slightly higher attenuation that enhances with contrast due to the increased vascularity of the abscess wall (Urol Clin North Am 1983;9:185; Radiology 1979;13:171)

Rx: Traditional rx is open or percutaneous drainage and abx (Urology 1985;25:142; J Urol 1982;127:425). In select cases, iv abx and observation may be all that is necessary (J Urol 1984;132:718; Arch IM 1980;140:914). If hematogenous spread is suspected, a penicillinase-resistant penicillin should be used (Ann IM 1977;87:305). Those assoc with gram negatives are treated with ampicillin plus aminoglycoside pending culture results

2.4 RENAL AND URETERAL TUBERCULOSIS

Cause: *Mycobacterium tuberculosis*, blood-borne mets. Previous lung infection may occur many yr prior to renal/ureteral disease

Epidem: Male:female ratio 2:1; most pts 20–40 yr, but increase incidence among pts 45–55 yr and among pts >70 yr. Autopsy study of pulmonary TB revealed unsuspected renal foci in 73% of cases, usually bilateral (Am Rev Respir Dis 1975;111:647). Most common site of ureteral involvement is distal ureter at UVJ

Pathophys: Blood-borne. Bacteria settle in blood vessels, typically near glomeruli. Depending on dose of infecting organism, virulence of organism and host resistance, tubercles may be replaced by fibrous tissue or continue to multiply and coalesce leading to caseous necrosis

Sx: Flank pain if obstructed

Si: Abnl chest xray, calcifications in kidneys on plain film of abdomen, back pain, flank pain

Crs: May lead to calyceal strictures, calyceal destruction, UPJO, TB interstitial nephritis, abscess formation, UVJ obstruction

Cmplc: Renal failure (Tubercle 1990;71:5), HT (J Urol 1980;123:822)

Lab: UA, c + s sterile pyuria (typically >20 wbc/hpf) common, but superimposed infection is present in 20% (Campbell's Urology 1998,7(24):807–836). Microscopic hematuria and intermittent gross hematuria may occur. Culture of 3 morning urine specimens for mycobacteria establishes dx in 80–90% of cases (Principles and Practice of Infectious Disease 2000;5:2602). PPD: A positive reaction indicates that patient has been infected, provided pt has not been vaccinated with BCG; but can't be regarded as indication of active TB

Xray: KUB may show calcification in areas of kidney or lower urinary tract. IVP: Renal lesions may appear as distorted calyx (occluded, destroyed or deformed). Rarely, affected kidney may not function. Ureteric involvement including stricture disease may be identified. IVP superior to CT

Rx: Chemotherapy: 2 mo rifampin (450–600 mg/d), isoniazide (300 mg/d), pyrazinamide (25 mg/kg body weight/d), ± streptomycin (1.0 gm if >50 kg body weight/d) then rifampin (600–900 mg/d 2–3 times/wk) and isoniazide (600 mg/d 2–3 times/wk) for 2–4 mo (Campbell's Urology 1998;7(24):807–836). Pts should be followed regularly after chemotherapy at 3, 6, 9, 12 mo with urine culture and IVP. If small calcifications present, then yearly KUB to follow the size of these. Surgical intervention indicated for large calcifications, nonfunctioning kidney with extensive calcification, and stricture disease (J Urol 1980;124:187; J Urol 1980;123:822)

2.5 XANTHOGRANULOMATOUS PYELONEPHRITIS (XGP)

Cause: Rare, severe, chronic renal infection that typically results in diffuse destruction of the renal tissue. Occurs in setting of obstruction and infection. *Proteus* is most common organism

Epidem: Most cases are unilateral. Found in 0.6–1.4% pts with renal inflammation evaluated pathologically (BJU 1972;44:296; Am J Clin Pathol 1955;25:1043). Peak incidence is in pts in their 50s to 70s. Female-to-male ratio of 3:1. 15% have DM

Pathophys: Thought to start with obstruction (stone or sloughed papilla) followed by infection that leads to destruction of tissue and deposition of lipid material by histiocytes. Granulomatous process then occurs. Xanthoma cells: lipid-laden macrophages. May affect kidney alone or progress to involve perinephric fat and retroperitoneum

Sx: Flank tenderness, malaise

Si: Fever, chills, flank pain, palpable flank mass, urgency, frequency, dysuria

Crs: May be treated with drainage but may progress to involve entire kidney, requiring nephrectomy

Cmplc: TCC, RCC (See 2.19 and 2.22), and squamous cell carcinoma of the pelvis have occurred with XGP (J Urol 1981;125:398; J Urol 1981;126:437; J Urol 1980;124:125)

DiffDx: Renal mass

Lab: UA, c + s; CBC may demonstrate anemia; hepatic dysfunction in up to 50% of pts (J Urol 1978;119:589)

Xray: IVP: Renal calculus identified in 38–70%, lack of excretion in 27–80%, and calyceal deformity in 46% (J Urol 1978;119:589). CT scan is most useful radiologic test, as it demonstrates large reniform mass with nondilated pelvis with central calcification. Renal parenchyma is replaced with fluid-filled masses that represent the dilated calyces and abscess cavities

Rx: If cannot r/o malignancy, nephrectomy is indicated. If disease is extensive, nephrectomy and removal of perinephric fat are warranted. If drainage alone is employed, condition may continue and develop a renal cutaneous fistula

2.6 MALACOPLAKIA

BJU 1999;84:464; Clin Infec Dis 1994;18:704; Am J Kidney Dis 1993;22:243

Cause: Exact etiology unknown. Condition appears to be related to abnormal intracellular killing by phagocytes, particularly macrophages. Localized to GU tract (58% of cases), bladder (40%), prostate, kidney (16%), ureter (11%), renal pelvis (10%), and testes. May be noted in other sites incl skin, vulva, vagina, adrenal, cerebrum, lungs, verterbrae, endometrium, pleura, gluteal muscles, tonsils, conjunctiva, spleen, hip joint (J Urol 1981;125:139)

Epidem: Female-to-male ratio of 4:1. Peak incidence is after age 50 yr (BJU 1982;54:181). 80–90% of pts have persistent UTI, *E. coli* being most commonly identified organism (70%) (J Pathol 1983;140:275; J Urol 1981;125:139). 40% of pts have intercurrent systemic illness, carcinoma, AIDS, or autoimmune disease (Urol Radiol 1990;12:157). Bilateral renal involvement in 64% of pts with renal disease

Pathophys: Thought to be related to defective lysosomes and abnormal microtubular assembly. May reflect alterations in cGMP and AMP levels (BJU 1999;84:464). Pathognomonic dx of malacoplakia are intracytoplasmic and extracytoplasmic inclusions, Michaelis–Gutman bodies. Calcium phosphate crystals and iron are main components of the Michaelis–Gutman body. Dx confirmed by histopathology

Sx: Bladder (frequency, urgency, dysuria), prostate (obstructive voiding symptoms), and renal (flank pain, N/V, abdominal pain)

Si: Prostate (firm, enlarged prostate, elevated PSA), renal (fever, palpable mass), testes (palpable intratesticular mass), 70% are fluctuant (Am J Clin Pathol 1967;47:135)

Crs: If untreated, may progress to large fungating mass; if in ureter, may lead to obstruction and loss of renal function

Cmplc: Mortality can exceed 50% (J Urol 198;125:139)

DiffDx: Renal (megalocystic interstitial nephritis, xanthogranulomatous pyelonephritis, lymphoma, amyloidosis, pyelonephritis, glomerulonephritis, vasculitis, renal vein thrombosis); bladder (bladder cancer); prostate (prostate cancer); ureter (ureteritis cystica)

Lab: UA: Hematuria, pyuria, bacteriuria. Urine culture. CBC: Anemia present in 82% of cases, elevated wbc in 60% (Am J Kidney Dis 193;22:243). Increased PSA may be present with prostatic involvement

Xray:

Renal Disease: IVP: Renal enlargement, lack of function, presence of a mass or hydronephrosis (Br J Radiol 1985;58:175; Nejm 1978;229:1110). US demonstrates multiple irregular masses, renal enlargement, distorted echogenicity (J Urol 1992;147:115; Br J Radiol 1985;58:175; Br J Radiol 1984;57:751). CT demonstrates poor enhancement, lack of excretion, renal enlargement, multiple mildly enhancing heterogeneous solid masses (J Urol 1992;147:115; Am J Nephrol 1990;10:416; Radiology 1980;136:33)

Bladder: IVP may demonstrate filling defect in bladder. CT demonstrates circumferential bladder wall thickening, multiple lobules, large masses (J Comput Assist Tomogr 1985;9:119; J Comput Assist Tomogr 1983;7:541)

Ureteral: IVP may appear similar to pyeloureteritis cystica or multiple TCC of the ureter; proximal ureteral dilation may be present (Am J Roentgenol 1972;116:830)

Testes: US demonstrates testicular mass that cannot be distinguished from neoplasm (J Urol 1998;159:508)

Rx: Mainstay of rx is long-term abx. Quinolones effective in 80–90% of pts. Other agents such as Tm/S, which assist intracellular killing of bacteria, may be used. In select studies, vitamin C and bethanechol have been helpful in controlling the disease by increasing cGMP–cAMP ratio, which improves macrophage function (J Urol 1979;122:703; Nejm 1977;279:1413). For unilateral renal disease, nephrectomy is often necessary, as disease tends to be more aggressive. In testis, rx is orchiectomy in addition to abx. In prostatic disease, confirmed by bx, treat with abx and vitamin C for up to 6 mo. If the PSA was elevated, expect it to decrease with effective rx. For bladder, TUR of the lesion in addition to abx. In ureteral disease, successful rx with stenting and abx has been reported (BJU 1987;59:485). D/c or taper immunosuppressive rx whenever possible in the rx of malacoplakia in immunocompromised pts

2.7 COCCIDIOIDOMYCOSIS

Nejm 1995;532:1077

Cause: *Coccidioides immitis*

Epidem: Airborne spread (inhalation) of mycelial-stage infective spores; endospore spread in body (Nejm 1979;301:358). American Southwest: Worst in wet season, especially if exposed to dirt in spring and late fall. Increased prevalence in DM, steroid use, AIDS, immunocompromised

Pathophys: Postmortem studies: Involvement of kidney in 35–60%, adrenal in 16–32%, prostate in 6% (J Urol 1988;140:370) of those with disseminated disease. Coccidioidal cystitis rare. Prostate one of more common GU sites, scrotal infection may occur

Sx: That of disseminated disease

Si: Boggy or indurated prostate, scrotal swelling, indurated epididymis, draining sinus

Crs: GU involvement is manifestation of multiorgan disease

Lab: c + s of draining sinus; tissue bx: stain with periodic acid–Schiff or methenamine silver to identify coccidioidal spherule; prostate secretions often pos if prostate involved (Ann IM 1976;85:34); urine c + s may be pos. Serol: Comp-fix ab titer >1/16 suggests disseminated active disease. Pos in 14/15 (Nejm 1970;283:326), decreases with successful rx. Counterimmunoelectrophoresis has 8% false-neg rate (Ann IM 1976;85:740). Skin test: 20–50% false neg (Am Rev Respir Dis 1988;138:1081); indicates present or past disease

Xray: IVP: If kidney involved may look similar to TB with motheaten calyces, infundibular stenosis, and renal calcifications (J Urol 1995;113:82)

Rx: Isolated lesions, such as epididymal lesions, may be treated with excision alone; otherwise in setting of systemic disease, iv amphotericin B (500–2500 mg total dose)

2.8 HISTOPLASMOSIS

Cause: *Histoplasma capsulatum*

Epidem: Bat and bird vectors via airborne spores. Midwest and southern U.S.

Pathophys: GU tract may be involved in disseminated infection; adrenal affected in 82%, kidney in 18%, prostate in 6% (Am J Med 1959;27:278). Penile ulcers and epididymal infection may occur with disseminated disease. Conjugal transmission

Sx: Obstructive voiding symptoms with prostatic infection

Si: Those of disseminated disease; if epididymis involved, may be indurated or fluctuant

Lab: c + s of sputum, gastric washings or abscess may be (+); tissue bx may reveal organism with methamine silver. With disseminated disease, peripheral blood smears may show intraleukocytic budding yeast (Jama 1985;253:3148)

Hem: Anemia, thrombocytopenia, marrow culture and stain (+) (all only in disseminated disease)

Serol: (Ann IM 1982;97:680). Comp-fix ab titer (+) in 96% of patients with active, disseminated disease. Immunodiffusion ab titer (+) in 87%, RIA for ag pos in urine (90%) and blood (50%)

in disseminated disease (Nejm 1986;314:83) and more accurate than ab titers (Ann IM 1991;115: 936)

Skin test: Many false pos and neg, interfere with serologic testing (Am Rev Respir Dis 1964; 90:927)

Rx: Systemic amphotericin B: 1/2 mg/kg body weight iv × 2/wk to total of 35–40 mg/kg body weight initial course (Ann IM 1971;75:511); use prophylactically if hx and starting steroids (Nejm 1969;280:2060) or if pt has AIDS and has been treated to cure (Ann IM 1989;111:655). Ketoconazole 400 mg qd × 6 mo cures 85% (Ann IM 1985;103:861) or itraconazole (Sporanox) 200 mg po bid, prevents relapse in AIDS pts (Ann IM 1993;118:610)

2.9 ASPERGILLUS

Cause: Fungal infection with *Aspergillus fumigatus, A. flavus, A. niger.* Aspergilli found in soil, decomposing vegetation, paint, chemical agents, medication bottles, refrigerators, bird excreta

Epidem: Second to candida as opportunistic organism in pts with malignancy, DM, immunosuppression. Seen in those with IV drug abuse and AIDS. Kidney involved in 13% of cases (Medicine 1970;49:147)

Sx: Flank pain, tenderness

Si: Fever

Lab: Urine fungal cx or tissue bx: Fungus demonstrated with methenamine silver or periodic acid–Schiff stain. PCR amplification helps detect *Aspergillus* in blood and urine (Mol Cell Probes 1993;7:121)

Xray: IVP may show filling defects in collecting system or ureter

Rx: IV amphotericin B or itraconazole. Rarely, nephrectomy

2.10 CRYPTOCOCCOSIS

Cause: In GU tract, *Cryptococcus neoformans*

Epidem: Ubiquitous fungus. Airborne, birds (pigeons) probable vector, grows in bird guano. Worldwide. Increased incidence in immunocompromised and AIDS pts

Pathophys: May affect adrenal, kidney, prostate, penis. In those with AIDS, prostate is reservoir for cryptococcus after rx of cryptococcal meningitis (Ann IM 1989;111:125)

Si: Renal abscess: Hematuria, pyuria, proteinuria. Prostatic abscess: Urinary retention, voiding difficulties. Penis: May have exophytic mass (J Infect Dis 1988;158:897)

Lab: Urine c + s: With renal infections only 40% (+) urine cx (J Urol 1973;109:695). Tissue bx for cx and stain

Rx: Renal involvement: iv amphotericin, poor prognosis. Prostate: Fluconazole 200–600 mg/d (Ann IM 1991;115:285), dose and length of rx not well defined. Penile: Excisional bx, amphotericin B (1 gm) and 5-FC (100 mg/kg body wt for 6 wk)

2.11 BLASTOMYCOSIS

Nejm 1986;314:529

Cause: *Blastomyces dermatitidis*

Epidem: Airborne in rotten wood dust. Great Lakes and Southeastern U.S.

Pathophys: GU involvement in 15–30% pts with systemic disease (J Urol 1983;130:160; J Urol 1975;113:650; J Urol 1969;102:754). Epididymis affected in 91%, prostate in 73%, kidney in 9%, prepuce in 9% (J Urol 1975;113:650). May also affect adrenal

Sx: Frequency, hesitancy, urinary retention

Si: Epididymal induration, nocturia, large fluctuant prostate

Crs: GU blastomycosis is a manifestation of systemic disease

Lab:
  Skin Test: Pos in <40% proven cases (Am Rev Respir Dis 1988;138:1081; Nejm 1986;314:529)

Serol: CF ab (+) in only 10% (Nejm 1974;290:540); immunodiffusion (+) in 28% of true (+); enzyme immunoassay (+) in 77%

Tissue: Fungal stain "broad-neck" yeast forms in infected tissue

Xray: C-xray (+) if pulmonary involvement

Rx: GU blastomycosis requires systemic amphotericin B in doses of 1–3 gm (J Urol 1983;130:160; J Urol 1975;113:650). Ketoconazole (400 mg/d) has been effective in cutaneous and prostatic infections (J Urol 1983;130:160)

2.12 RETROPERITONEAL FIBROSIS

Cause: Proposed causes include retroperitoneal hemorrhage, urinary extravasation, trauma, perianeurysmal inflammation, XRT, surgery, inflammatory bowel disease, collagen disease, fat necrosis, malignancy, infections, methysergide (Sansert)-induced (BMJ 1988;296:240; Can J Surg 1984;27:111; Surgery 1977;81:250)

Epidem: Incidence is 1 in 200,000 (Eur Urol 1982;8:45). Average age at onset of sx is 50 yr, with 70% of pts ages 30–60 (NY State J Med 1989;89:511). Uncommon in childhood, idiopathic in 2/3 of cases, males > females. Bilateral ureteral involvement present in 2/3 of adult cases (Pediatr Radiol 1988;18:245)

Pathophys: In setting of abdominal aortic aneurysms, retroperitoneal fibrosis is thought to be secondary to a hypersensitivity reaction to antigens leaking into retroperitoneum from atheromatous plaques (BMJ 1988;297:240). Fibrous process envelopes ureter and tends to drag middle third of the ureter medially. On histologic evaluation, primary finding is collagen fibers and fibroblasts (Campbell's Urology 1998;7(10):387)

Sx: May be related to entrapment and compression of the ureters, inferior vena cava, aorta and its branches, or gonadal vessels

Si: Oliguria, anuria, renal insufficiency, lower-extremity edema, weight loss, fatigue, mild fever

Crs: If untreated, renal function may be lost; 1/3 of pts have nonfunctioning kidney on presentation

Cmplc: Loss of renal function

DiffDx: Malignant adenopathy, lymphoma, amyloidosis, retroperitoneal hematoma, cervical carcinoma, pancreatic carcinoma, sarcoma, multiple myeloma

Lab: Elevated ESR in 94% (J Urol 1979;122:1), serum electrolytes, BUN, creatinine levels

Xray: CT scan is most definitive study for dx and to determine extent of retroperitoneal fibrosis (Urol Radiol 1982;4:95). IVP demonstrates smooth extrinsic narrowing of one or both ureters at level of L-S spine with proximal dilation. Ureters deviate medially at L3 or L4 (Am J Radiol 1973;119:812)

Rx: Varies with etiology. R/o malignancy. If Sansert-related, condition will often regress with d/c of Sansert. For idiopathic retroperitoneal fibrosis rx is bilateral ureterolysis with or without steroid therapy, even in the presence of unilateral disease. Long-term success rate with surgical rx is 90% (Can J Surg 1984;27:111)

2.13 RENAL ADENOMA

Cause: Benign neoplasm <3 cm possible distal tubular epithelial origin (Semin Urol 1990;8:31)

Epidem: ? Truly benign lesion (J Urol 1970;103:31) versus malignant (Atlas of Tumor Pathology, 2nd series, fascicle 12. Washington, DC: Armed Forces Institute of Pathology, 1975). Considered RCC until proven otherwise (Urol Clin North Am 1993;20:193)

Pathophys: Histopath: Uniform basophilic or acidophilic cells without mitotic activity or cellular atypia (Campbell's Urology 1998;7(3):2283–2326)

Sx: Asx

Si: Incidental finding; may develop hematuria if erodes collecting system or adjacent vessels

DiffDx: RCC

Xray:

  CT: Similar appearance to renal cell carcinoma except for lack of calcification

Angio: Does not have AV fistulas or venous pooling seen with renal cell carcinoma

Rx: Surgical excision, ? partial nephrectomy, ? tendency for multicentricity

2.14 RENAL ONCOCYTOMA

Cause: Benign neoplasm of the kidney

Epidem: Exact incidence unknown. Approximately 3–7% of solid renal masses previously classified as RCC are now thought to be renal oncocytomas (Urol Clin North Am 1993;20:355). Males > females. Masses vary in size and may be large (median: 6 cm diameter). Typically unifocal and often an incidental finding

Pathophys: Characterized by histologic pattern of large eosinophilic cells with granular cytoplasm and polygonal form. Nuclei are low grade and mitoses are rare. They are thought to originate from distal renal tubules (collecting duct) (Virchows Arch 1987;52:375)

Sx: Asx but infrequently can be a cause of pain

Si: Hematuria and flank mass

Crs: Benign lesions

DiffDx: RCC

Lab: Not routinely indicated

Xray: Characteristic central scar may be identified on CT and MRI, and sometimes on US. Typical renal angiogram finding is a spoke-wheel or stellate pattern seldom associated with venous pooling or arteriovenous fistulae (Urol Radiol 1998;2:229). Typical angiographic picture is not always identified and there are no typical CT scan findings or specific radionuclide scans to reliably distinguish oncocytoma from renal cell carcinoma

Rx: Influenced by (1) the lack of a reliable x-ray study to differentiate RCC from oncocytoma and (2) presence of malignant cells and oncocytoma cells in same tumor. For relatively young healthy pts with tumors <4 cm, well encapsulated by CT, and confined to one pole of the kidney, renal exploration and partial nephrectomy may be considered. In elderly, high-risk patients, close observation may be indicated

2.15 RENAL ANGIOMYOLIPOMA (HAMARTOMA)

Cause: Benign renal tumor

Epidem: May occur as isolated phenomenon or as part of the syndrome assoc with tuberous sclerosis. 50% of those with angiomyolipoma have some or all of the stigmata of tuberous sclerosis. Screen all tuberous sclerosis pts for angiomyolipoma (J Urol 1987;138:477). Frequently bilateral, may be multiple and often large

Pathophys: Three primary histologic components: Unusual abdominal blood vessels, clusters of adipocytes, and sheets of smooth muscle

Sx: Often asx. If large, may cause local discomfort and GI sx by compressing the duodenum and stomach. Sudden increased pain may be related to spontaneous bleed

Si: Hypotension may be secondary to bleed within the lesion

Crs: Propensity for hemorrhage

Cmplc: Acute hemorrhage

DiffDx: In routine cases, hx and radiologic findings discern from other solid renal masses. If lesion cannot be discerned reliably, it should be removed (J Urol 1988;139:20)

Lab: Hgb and crit if severe pain/hypotension

Xray: CT preferred imaging modality (Am J Radiol 1988;151:497). Presence of fat within lesion is characteristic for angiomyolipoma

Rx: Controversial. For asx lesions <4 cm, lesion may be monitored annually by CT or US (J Urol 1986;135:1211). Larger lesions should be monitored semiannually (J Urol 1993;150:1782). If lesion size is increasing, embolization or renal-sparing surgery should be considered. Large angiomyolipomas assoc with severe sx are best treated with immediate selective arterial embolization if possible, or conservative renal-sparing surgery if embolization is not possible. In the setting of an acute bleed, embolization is first choice. With larger lesions, embolization is not successful and surgical excision is necessary

DISEASES OF THE KIDNEY AND URETER

2.16 RENAL LIPOMA

J Urol 1971;100:503

Cause: Probably originates from fat cells with the renal ᴄ ᴘsule or parenchyma

Epidem: Rare; noted in middle-aged women

Pathophys: Malignant potential suggested but not proven; confined within renal capsule

Sx: Flank pain

Si: Large renal mass, ± hematuria

Xray: CT: Fatty renal mass confined within the capsule

Rx: Surgical excision, usually via nephrectomy

2.17 JUXTAGLOMERULAR CELL TUMORS OF THE KIDNEY

Cause: Benign neoplasm of juxtaglomerular cell origin

Epidem: Increasing recognition of these tumors. Occurs in young pts (mean age 24 yr) (J Urol 1985;134:334). Female:male ratio of 1.7:1 (J Urol 1989;142:1560). Average size 2.5 cm, most ≤5 cm (J Urol 1985;134:334)

Pathophys: Juxtaglomerular apparatus consists of 3 components: mesangial cells, macula densa, and granular cells that contain renin. Hallmark of juxtaglomerular cell tumors is cells with secretory granules that contain renin, which stain deep blue to purple by Bowie method (Stain Technol 1966;41:291)

Sx: Blurry vision, HA, nocturia

Si: Marked HT (mean diastolic BP 142) (Arch IM 1972;130:682; Ann IM 1971;75:725), easy fatigability, nocturia

Cmplc: Hypertensive retinopathy (Am J Med 1967;43:963) and cmplc related to HT

DiffDx: RCC (Arch IM 1975;135:859), renal cyst (Am J Med 1976;61:579), Wilms' tumor (Lancet 1992;1:1180), pheo (J Ped 1976;89:950), hemangiopericytoma (Urology 1982;20:191), renal artery stenosis

Lab: Elevated peripheral plasma renin. Hypokalemia often present (J Urol 1989;142:1560; J Urol 1985;134:334). 24-h urine excretion steroids usually not elevated, but mild elevation above normal of urinary VMA and urine catecholamines has been reported (Cancer 1984;53:516). Renal vein renin levels may be helpful in lateralizing the side of tumor (J Urol 1985;134:334). Segmental renal vein sampling may reveal increased ratios not apparent with main renal vein sampling (J Peds 1979;94:247; Nephron 1978;21:325; Am J Med 1973;55:86)

Xray: Renal artery angiography reveals a hypovascular mass and eliminates renal artery stenosis. CT demonstrates tumor but cannot distinguish from other renal tumors (J Urol 1989;142:1560)

Rx: Surgical excision: Partial or total nephrectomy depending on size and location of lesion

DISEASES OF THE KIDNEY AND URETER

2.18 FIBROEPITHELIAL POLYP

Cause: Benign neoplasm. May be congenital (Radiology 1979;130:73) or secondary to chronic infection/irritation (Urology 1994;44:582; Urology 1980;16:355)

Epidem: 80% occur in boys; 70% on left side; 62% at UPJ, remainder distributed in order of frequency in posterior urethra, distal and mid ureter (J Urol 1986;136:476). Account for 0.5–4% of hydroureteronephrosis in children (J Urol 1997;158:569). Can occur at any age; male: female ratio of 3:2 (BJU 1980;52:253). Usually length is 20–50 mm, but may be as long as 135 mm (BJU 1988;61:461). Most common benign neoplasm of ureter

Pathophys: Pathology: Core of mesodermal tissue covered by normal epithelium, may be cylindrical or sessile with multiple fronds

Sx: Flank pain, frequency, dysuria

Si: Hematuria, hydronephrosis

Cmplc: Rarely assoc with TCC (Urology 1994;44:582; J Urol 1976;115:651). May occur in assoc with calculi (J Urol 1989;142:1563)

Lab: Urine cytology to r/o TCC

Xray: IVP demonstrates a mobile, smooth, sharply demarcated, filiform filling defect. CT ureteroscopy useful to identify ureteral tumors (sens 81%, specif 100%). Identification of a stalk is most helpful in distinguishing fibroepithelial polyp from ureteral carcinoma

(J Urol 2000;163:42). Retrograde ureterography will also demonstrate an intraluminal filling defect

Rx: Endoscopic TUR for urethral polyps. Ureteroscopy and bx to confirm dx. Ureteral polyps may be removed endoscopically if stalk is identifiable; less commonly, open excision indicated. No recurrences have been noted with complete excision

---

2.19 RENAL CELL CARCINOMA (RCC)

Nejm 1996;335:865; Semin Oncol 2000;27(a):160; Curr Opin Urol 2000;12(3):260

Cause: Neoplasm of the renal parenchyma

Epidem: Accounts for 2% of all cancers; is the 7th leading cause of cancer. Male:female 2:1. Whites = blacks. Occurs predominantly in the 7th and 8th decades of life. Incidence increasing as is survival rate. 25–40% of cases are detected incidentally. 1/3 of cases have mets at presentation and 50% of those resected for cure are expected to relapse during course of disease (Semin Oncol 1989 (suppl);16:3). Common sites of mets: lung, bone, liver, adrenal, brain

Pathophys: RCC accounts for 80–85% of malignant renal tumors. Risk factors: Smoking, obesity, HT, rx for HT, unopposed estrogen therapy, occupational exposure to petroleum products, heavy metals and asbestos (Int J Cancer 1995;61:192; 1986;77:351; JNCI 1984;72:275). Rare familial forms of RCC present at a younger age, are autosomal dominant in inheritance, and typically have bilateral and multifocal tumors (Medicine 1989;68:1; Nejm 1979;301:592). Von Hippel–Lindau disease is a familial multiple cancer syndrome with increased risk of a variety of neoplasms incl RCC (40%) and renal cysts, retinal hemangiomas, hemangioblastomas of cerebellum and spinal cord, pheo and pancreatic carcinoma and cysts (Medicine 1989;68:1). Five histopathologic types of RCC identified:

Clear cell carcinoma (75–85% of tumors): Assoc with deletion of one or both copies of chromosome p (Cancer Res 1991;51:1544)

Chromophilic (papillary) (14% tumors): Usually small tumors; often multifocal and bilateral. Assoc with monosomy Y, trisomy 7 and 17 (Genes Chromosom Cancer 1991;3:249; Cancer 1976;38:2469)

Chromophobic (4%): Excellent prognosis; assoc with hypodiploid number of chromosomes and multiple chromosome losses but not 3p (Am J Surg Pathol 1995;19:1245; Genes Chromosom Cancer 1992;4:267)

Oncocytic: Rarely assoc with mets (J Urol 1993;150:295)

Collecting duct (Bellini's duct) tumor: Rare, clinically aggressive (Hum Pathol 1990;21:449)

Paraneoplastic syndromes present in <5% pts and include erythrocytosis, hepatic dysfunction (Stauffer's syndrome), amyloidosis (Semin Oncol 1983;10:390)

Prognostic indicators: Pathologic stage is foremost. Others include histologic pattern, nuclear grade, and DNA content (Urol Clin North Am 1993;20:247)

Staging system: Robson is used most frequently in U.S. TNM is also used. Robson (J Urol 1963;89:37):

I   Small, confined to capsule, min caliceal distortion
I   Large, confined to capsule, caliceal distortion
II   Ext to perirenal fat or ipsilat adrenal within Gerota's
IIIa Renal vein involvement
IIIa Renal vein and vena caval involvement
IIIa Vena caval involvement above diaphragm
IIIb Single ipsilat node involved
IIIb Mult regional, contralateral, or bilat nodes involved
IIIb Fixed regional nodes
IIIb Juxtaregional nodes involved
IIIc Combination of IIIa and IIIb
IVa Spread to contiguous organs except ipsilat adrenal
IVb Distant metastases

Sx: Abdominal pain (40%), malaise (Semin Oncol 1983;10:390)

Si: Palpable flank or abdominal mass (30–40%), hematuria (50–60%), fever, night sweats, weight loss, new-onset varicocele

DiffDx: Renal cyst, renal adenoma, oncocytoma

Lab: CBC, lytes, BUN and creatinine, glucose, alkaline phosphatase

Xray: Chest xray to r/o lung mets. Tumors ≤3 cm: Sens of urography, US, and CT are 67, 79, and 94%, respectively (Radiology 1988;166:637). CT for staging has 90% accuracy (Am J Roentgenol 1987;148:59). MRI with IV gadolinium superior to CT in evaluating IVC when tumor involvement is suspect; also useful in pt with contrast allergy or renal insufficiency (Radiology

1991;180:85). Bone scan to r/o bone mets if alkaline phosphatase elevated

Rx: Surgical rx is the main rx for RCC; typically involves removal of kidney and surrounding Gerota's fascia, surrounding lymph nodes, and in the setting of the upper pole tumor, the ipsilateral adrenal gland. Nephron-sparing surgery (partial nephrectomy) indicated for pts with solitary kidney, bilateral tumors, and in select pts in whom the contralateral kidney is threatened by assoc disease process such as HT and DM. Local recurrence rate with partial nephrectomy is 4–10% (Urology 1994;43:160; J Urol 1994;152:39; 1993;150:319; 1992;148:24; 1990;144:852; 1989;141:835). Partial nephrectomy may also be considered in pts with small (<4 cm) polar lesions with a normal contralateral kidney. Systemic rx for advanced disease: Hormonal rx and chemotherapy have had little to no effect on RCC (Semin Oncol 1995;22:42). Biologic response modifiers yield better results and include interferon-alpha (objective response up to 30% in select patients) (J Clin Oncol 1991;9:832) and interleuken-2 with response rates 13.5–18.6%, varying with method of administration (J Urol 1999;161:381). Combination therapy and tumor vaccines also being evaluated

2.20 RENAL SARCOMAS

Cause: Malignant neoplasm of kidney
Epidem: 1–3% of malignant renal tumors, increase in incidence with age (Am Surgeon 1995;61:456; Tokai J Exp Clin Med 1982;7:365), female:male 1.4:1 (BJU 1971;43:546), 40–60 years of age, rarely bilateral
Pathophys: Leiomyosarcoma accounts for 60% of renal sarcomas. Most arise from renal capsule or pericapsular tissue, but may arise from muscle fibers in renal pelvis or in wall of renal vessels (Br J Urol 1971;43:546). Other lesions include liposarcoma (19% of renal sarcomas) and osteosarcoma (very rare)
Sx: Flank pain, GI sx
Si: Flank mass, ± hematuria, weight loss
Crs: Poor prognosis. Leiomyosarcoma mets to lungs, bone, liver, mesentery (J Urol 1973;100:974)

DiffDx: Other renal tumors including RCC

Lab: UA may demonstrate hematuria

Xray:

> *CT:* With leiomyosarcoma, tumor tends to displace and compress kidney; fat density seen with liposarcoma and bone may be seen in osteosarcoma

> *Angio:* Hypovascular tumor without arteriovenous fistulas (Radiology 1987;162:353)

Rx: Leiomyosarcoma: Radical nephrectomy; early local and distal recurrence common (BJU 1991;68:659). Some response with advanced, metastatic, or unresectable disease to ifosfamide-based regimens (J Clin Oncol 1993;12:230; J Clin Oncol 1989;7:1208). Osteogenic sarcoma and liposarcoma best treated with radical nephrectomy

2.21 SECONDARY TUMORS OF THE KIDNEY

Cause: Metastatic lesions

Epidem: Kidney frequent site of metastases from both solid (J Urol 1971;105:492) and hematologic malignancies, most commonly lymphoma and lymphoblastoma. More commonly identified postmortem

Sx: Often asx, but may produce flank pain

Si: Hematuria

Xray:

> *CT:* (J Comput Assist Tomogr 1983;7:245). Often incidental CT finding. CT guided bx helpful to determine primary if unknown or uncertain and to r/o RCC

> *Angio:* Mets to kidney are often round and hypovascular, lacking the neovascularity often seen with RCC

Rx: As per primary malignancy

2.22 TRANSITIONAL CELL CARCINOMA (TCC) OF RENAL PELVIS AND URETER

Cause: Malignant neoplasm

Epidem: Renal pelvic tumors account for 10% of all renal tumors. TCC accounts for 90% of upper tract tumors (J Urol 1980;123:357). Ureteral tumors: Male:female 3:1, whites:blacks 2:1 (Ann Cancer Stat Rev 1987; NIH pub no. 88–2789). Peak incidence in 50s to 70s (J Urol 1989;142:280). Increased incidence with Balkan endemic nephropathy (J Urol 1975;114:858) and cigarette smokers. Other possible causes incl analgesics, coffee consumption, cyclophosphamide, occupational carcinogens, inflammation secondary to stones and UTIs, familial cancer syndromes (Arch Pathol Lab Med 1993;117:1156; BJU 1993;72:177; Cancer Res 1992;52:254; Int J Cancer 1989;44:965; Cancer Res 1989;49:1045; J Urol 1987;137:1226; Kidney Int 1986;30:81)

Pathophys: Ureteral tumors: Most common in distal ureter (73%) (J Urol 1980;123:357)

Si: Gross or microscopic hematuria in 75% (J Urol 1981;135:25; 1970;103:590), hydronephrosis if lesion is obstructing

Sx: Flank pain (30%)

Crs: Upper tract TCC occurs in 2–4% of pts with bladder cancer (J Urol 1989;41:1311) and up to 13% in occupational hazard-related bladder cancer (J Urol 1988;140:745). 30–75% patients with upper tract TCC have bladder tumor at some time (J Urol 1989;142:280; Cancer 1988;62:2016; BJU 1988;61:198). TCC mets may occur by direct extension, hematogenous or lymphatic spread (Urology 1985;25:310)

Tumor grade and stage are most important prognostic variables. Low-grade tumor: median survival 67 mo; high-grade tumor: median survival 14 mo. Low stage: median survival 97 mo. High stage: median survival 13 mo (Cancer 1988;62:2016).

Despite new diagnostic modalities and treatments, the survival rate for ureteral cancer has failed to improve from the 1970s to 1980s (Urol Int 1997;58:13)

TNM staging (Spiessl B, Beahrs OH, Hermanek P, et al. Renal pelvis and ureter. In: Spiessl B, Beahrs OH, Hermanek P, et al., eds. UICC TNM Atlas Illustrated Guide to the TNM/p TNM

Classification of Malignant Tumours. Berlin: Springer-Verlag, 1989:260)

T Tis: Carcinoma in situ
    Ta: Epithelial confined, usually a papillary lesion
    T1: Tumor invades lamina propria
    T2: Tumor invades muscularis propria
    T3: Invasion of peripelvic/periureteral tissue or renal parenchyma
    T4: Involvement of contiguous organs
N N0: No nodal involvement
    N1: Only one pos node ≤2 cm
    N2: One pos node ≥2 cm to ≤5 cm or mult pos nodes <5 cm
    N3: Pos nodes >5 cm
M M0: No hematogenous or distant mets
    M1: Hematogenous or distant mets

Lab: UA may show microscopic hematuria. Urine cytology inaccurate with low-grade tumors

Xray: IVP: 50–75% of pts have a filling defect (J Urol 1981;135:25). DiffDx of filling defect: Overlying bowel gas, crossing vessel, blood clot, stone, sloughed renal papilla, fungal ball, fibroepithelial polyp, malacoplakia, TB. Retrograde studies: Visualize collecting system if IVP inadequate; 75% accuracy in establishing diagnosis of TCC of upper tracts (J Urol 1981;135:25). Brush bx: Sens 91%, specif 88%, accuracy 89% (Am J Radiol 1989;153:313). CT helpful in dx and staging; soft-tissue mass, average HU of 46, range 10–70 (Urol Clin North Am 1984;11:567). Cysto: r/o TCC bladder. Ureteroscopy helpful in dx, allows for bx

Rx:

Renal Pelvic Tumor: Nephroureterectomy including cuff of bladder
Proximal ureteral and midureteral tumors: If low grade, low stage: segmental resection and reapproximation; if multifocal or moderately to poorly differentiated, then nephroureterectomy with cuff of bladder
Distal Ureteral Tumors: Low grade without multifocal lesions: distal ureterectomy and ureteral reimplantation; high grade, multifocal: probably best served with nephroureterectomy with cuff of bladder

5-yr survival rates for nephroureterectomy plus cuff of bladder: Tis, Ta, T1, 91%; T2, 43%; T3 or T4, N1 or N2, 23%; and N3 or M1, 0% (Cancer 1975;35:1626)

2.23 UROLITHIASIS

Cause: Key event in stone formation is supersaturation. More common stone types include calcium oxalate (70–80%), cystine (1–5%), uric acid (5–10%), calcium phosphate (5–10%), and struvite (5–10%). Rare stones include ammonium acid urate, triamterene, and indinivir

Epidem: Prevalence of 2–3%. Recurrence rate is about 10% at 1 yr and 50% at 10 yr for calcium oxalate stones (Ann IM 1989;111:1006). Peak incidence of stones occurs in pts in their 20s to 40s (Miner Electrol Metab 1987;13:257). Male:female ratio 3:1 (Urol Clin North Am 1997;24: 97). Prevalence higher in mountainous, desert, and tropical areas and during the summer (J Urol 1956;75:209). Causes of stone formation include the following:

Hereditary disorders: familial renal tubular acidosis (RTA), cystinuria, xanthinuria, glucose 6-phosphate deficiency, hypoxanthine-guanine phosphoribosyl transferase deficiency, phosphoribosylpyrophosphate overactivity, oxaluria, dehydroxyadenineuria

Dietary excesses: vitamin C ingestion, oxalate, purines, calcium

Sedentary lifestyle or immobilization

Thiazide-induced

UTIs with urea-splitting organisms (eg, *Proteus*)

Myeloproliferative disorders

Gastrointestinal disorders (inflammatory bowel disease)

Dehydration

Hypercalcemic disorders: hyperparathyroidism, sarcoidosis, histoplasmosis, leprosy, hyperthyroidism, secondary to glucocorticoids, malignancy, tuberculosis, coccidiomycosis, silicosis, pheo

Pathophys: Key event is supersaturation in the urine followed by crystallization, which is dependent on urine pH, temperature, and concentration of the major urinary ions. Once crystallization occurs, aggregation and retention must occur for a calculus to form. Urine contains constituents, which may promote or inhibit stone formation. Inhibitors of stone formation include citrate, mg, nephrocalcin, Tamm–Horsfall mucoprotein. Anatomic abnl such as medullary sponge kidney, UPJO and UVJ obstruction can predispose to crystal retention

Sx: Flank pain, nausea, renal or ureteral colic

Si: Inability for pt to get comfortable, hematuria, pyuria, hydronephrosis, vomiting, urinary frequency, flank/abdominal tenderness. Fever not usually present unless there is a UTI

Crs: Majority of stones <4–5 mm will pass spontaneously. Obstructing ureteral stones >6 mm seldom pass spontaneously. May take up to 1 mo for small stone to pass. Rx indicated if pt is anuric, pain is not controlled with oral pain medications, stone is too large to pass spontaneously, and in the setting of a UTI

Cmplc: Prolonged obstruction can lead to loss of renal function, recurrent UTIs if stone is infected

DiffDx: Urothelial tumor, blood clot

Lab: First time stone former: Serial $Ca^{2+} \times 3$, serum K^+, CO_2, and Cl^-. Urine for pH and c + s and look for crystals. Recurrent stone or metabolically active stone disease (new stones or stones that are increasing in size): Check serum $Ca^{2+} \times 3$, serum K^+, CO_2, Cl^-, phosp, and PTH. Also, two 24-h urine collections to test for Ca^{2+}, oxalate, Mg^{2+}, citrate, Na^+, creatinine, and uric acid, in appropriate containers

Rx: Stone prevention: Hydration. Rx abnls present in 24-h urine studies. If serum Ca^{2+} level elevated, check PTH; if elevated, evaluate for hyperparathyroidism. In acute stone, rx varies with pt clinical status, size of stone, and stone location. If pt is asx or pain is controlled with oral pain medication or stone is small, rx is hydration, oral pain medication, and observe. If pt pain is poorly controlled and/or stone is large, rx varies with stone size and location. If obstruction and UTI, abx and decompression, either via ureteral stent or percutaneous nephrostomy indicated first, followed by rx of stone

Renal calculi: ESWL is ideal first-line rx except for staghorn stones, which usually require combination rx

Ureteral calculi: Distal ureteral calculi may be treated endoscopically. Proximal ureteral calculi may be rx with ESWL or endoscopy

Rarely is open stone surgery (pyelolithotomy or ureterolithotomy) performed at this time. Uric acid stones may rx medically. If patient has sx, an indwelling JJ stent may be placed until stone is dissolved

ESWL is unpredictable in its effect on cystine stones, and upper size limit is 3 cm (J Urol 1991;145:25)

See Table 2–1 for rx of various 24-h urine abnls

Actions of various rx agents are as follows:

Thiazides: Act on distal tubule to inhibit Na^+ reabsorption and augment Ca^{2+} reabsorption independently. Only effective if on Na^+-restricted diet. Side effects incl fatigue, impotence, muscle weakness, hypokalemia, hyperuricemia, hyperuricosuria, metabolic alkalosis

Sodium cellulose phosphate: Nonabsorbable ion exchange resin. Binds Ca^{2+}, preventing intestinal absorption. May bind Mg^{2+} also, so may need to replete. By binding Ca^{2+}, may increase amount of oxalate available for intestinal absorption

Orthophosphate (Neutra-Phos): Decreases serum 1,25-dihydroxyvitamin D levels and lowers urinary Ca^{2+} excretion. Also stimulates excretion of pyrophosphate and citrate. Side effects incl diarrhea and soft-tissue calcification

Allopurinol: Decreases serum and urinary uric acid levels. Side effects include skin rash and reversible elevations in liver function tests. If rash occurs, d/c medication immediately, as condition may progress to Stevens–Johnson syndrome

Pyridoxine: May decrease production of oxalate by enhancing conversion of glyoxylate to glycine

D-*penicillamine and Thiola:* Cystine-binding agents. Side effects include proteinuria with nephrotic syndrome, fevers, rash, thrombocytopenia, arthralgia, GI upset. Need to supplement with vitamin B6

Captopril: Appears to bind cystine and also have effect on renal tubule to decrease urinary cystine level (J Urol 1995;154:164; Am J Kidney Dis 1993;21:504)

Table 2-1. Urolithiasis

	Hypercalciuria	Hyperuricosuria	Hyperoxaluria	Cystinuria	Hypocitraturia	Hypomagnesuria
Definition	>4 mg/kg body wt/ 24-h, >300 mg/24-h for male, >275 mg/ 24-h for female	>600–700 mg/ 24-h urine	>40–50 mg/24-h urine	>400 mg/24-h urine	<300–320 mg/ 24-h urine (if <50 mg, it's RTA)	<50 mg/24-h urine
Type	*Absorptive (I&II):* Normal serum Ca²⁺, low PTH; type II, normal fasting urine Ca²⁺ *Renal leak:* Normal serum Ca²⁺, +/– high PTH, increased fasting urine Ca²⁺ *Resorptive:* High serum Ca²⁺, high PTH, high fasting urine Ca²⁺	70% dietary, 30% overproduction; hyperuricosuria may initiate calcium oxalate stone formation by epitaxy gouty diathesis: Acidic urine (pH <5.5) ± hyperuricosuria. Overproduction may be due to myeloproliferative dz, glycogen storage dz, malignancy, diarrhea	5 causes: overindulgence, excess vitamin C, endogenous production, primary hyperoxaluria, inflammatory bowel dz	Cystine solubility is pH dependent. Increased solubility with pH > 7.5	Citrate is a stone inhibitor; citrate excretion decreased by metabolic acidosis, hypokalemia, infections	Magnesium is an inhibitor of calcium crystallization
Ddx	Diff type I & II: low Ca²⁺, oxalate, Na⁺ diet for 1 wk, check 24-h urine; if urine Ca²⁺ >200 type I, <200 type II		45–60 mg/d: dietary 45–400 mg/d: endogenous 80–400 mg/d: inflammatory bowel dz			

Table 2–1. (cont'd)

	Hypercalciuria	Hyperuricosuria	Hyperoxaluria	Cystinuria	Hypocitraturia	Hypomagnesuria
	Diff type II from renal leak: 2-h urine for Ca^{2+} after 14–16 h, overnight fast: >30 mg Ca^{2+} is renal leak					
Prevention	Absorptive type I: Sodium cellulose phosphate + magnesium gluconate 1–1.5 gm bid and low-oxalate diet or thiazides (HydroDiuril 50 mg bid) and KCl. Absorptive type II: Diet restriction to 600 mg per day of Ca^{2+} and low-oxalate dietary ± thiazides or Neutra-Phos (500 mg tid or qid). Renal leak: Thiazides	Hyperuricosuric calcium oxalate stones: Allopurinol 300 mg/d, Na^+ restriction (150 mEq/d) or potassium citrate 60 mEq/d in 3 doses. Gouty diathesis: Alkalinize urine with sodium bicarbonate or potassium citrate to keep pH 7. Low-methionine diet	Dietary excess: Restrict primary hyperoxaluria: pyridoxine 800–1000 mg/d in divided doses and/or magnesium gluconate 500 mg bid; enteric: calcium 0.25–1 gm qid or cholestyramine 8–16 gm/d in divided doses	Alkalinize urine to pH 7.5 with potassium citrate 30–60 mEq/d in divided doses; D-penicillamine 2 gm in 4 divided doses, start at 250 mg/d, increase gradually, or Thiola 800 mg/d in 3 divided doses on empty stomach. Titrate Thiola and D-penicillamine to keep cystine <400 mg/d in urine. Captopril in isolated cases	Potassium citrate 60–120 mEq/d in divided doses or Neutra-Phos	Magnesium gluconate 500 mg po bid, magnesium oxide, or magnesium hydroxide

2.24 RENAL TRAUMA

Urol Clin North Am 1989;16:187

Cause: Blunt trauma from motor vehicle accidents, falls, blunt physical contact with external objects. Penetrating trauma from knife wounds, gunshot wounds, and other objects

Epidem: Preexisting renal abnls (UPJO) make renal injury more likely following trauma. Hx of sudden deceleration assoc with increased risk of renal trauma. Blunt trauma accounts for 90% of renal injuries. Renal injury present in about 10% of abdominal traumas

Pathophys: Blunt renal trauma results from shearing forces that exceed tensile strength of renal parenchyma. Deceleration or crush injuries may thrust kidney against ribcage, vertebrae, or solid object. Sudden deceleration may stretch renal artery and produce intimal tear, leading to subintimal dissection. In children with UPJOs, deceleration and hyperextension injuries may lead to UPJ disruption

Classification: Minor (70%): Superficial renal lacerations, renal contusions, small subcapsular hematomas. Major: Deep parenchymal lacerations into collecting system, renovascular pedicle injuries, shattered kidneys

Sx: Hypotension, abdominal pain

Si: Flank hematoma and hematuria (degree of hematuria does not predict degree of renal injury)

Crs: Minor renal trauma requires no surgical intervention. Shattered kidneys may cause life-threatening bleeding. Renal pedicle injuries require prompt identification and rx to salvage renal function. Major renal trauma, if blunt, rx depends on injury and other assoc injuries; major penetrating renal trauma requires surgical rx

Cmplc: Page kidney (a kidney compressed by a subcapsular or perinephric process, such as a hematoma, which causes renal ischemia) leading to renovascular HT, infection, bleeding

Lab: UA, c + s, CBC, electrolytes, BUN, creatinine

Xray: Renal imaging indicated with all penetrating trauma to the flank, back, or abdomen. In adult pts with blunt trauma, renal imaging indicated for gross hematuria or for microscopic hematuria if assoc with shock. CT provides greater sens and specif compared to IVP in detecting and characterizing renal injury (J Urol 1991;146:274; 1982;128:456)

Rx: Routine trauma care should be administered—the ABCs (airway, breathing, circulation). Rx varies with degree of injury. Minor trauma: Observation and bed rest until urine clears and vital signs are stable. Major trauma: Surgery indicated for uncontrolled bleeding, renovascular injury, nonviable parenchyma, major urinary extravasation. With surgical exploration there is an 18% nephrectomy rate for major renal trauma (J Trauma 1982;22:285). Renal trauma should be explored through midline incision and renal vessels exposed and controlled with vessel loops prior to opening Gerota's fascia. Devitalized tissue is debrided, tears in collecting system closed, and major vascular injuries repaired

2.25 URETERAL INJURY

Cause: External trauma or iatrogenic. Iatrogenic ureteral injury may occur with gynecologic procedures (hysterectomy, oophorectomy, bladder neck suspension), general surgical procedures (colectomy, appendectomy, vascular surgery), aortoiliac bypass surgery, urologic surgery (ureterolithotomy, pelvic laparoscopic procedures)

Epidem: Iatrogenic injury occurs most commonly at pelvic brim where ureter crosses iliac artery and where it courses posterior to broad ligament and ovarian vessels in females

Pathophys: Classification: (1) mechanism (blunt versus penetrating), (2) level of injury (proximal, mid, distal ureter), (3) from time of injury to recognition, (4) presence of assoc injuries (Urol Clin North Am 1989;16:237)

Sx: Abdominal and/or flank pain

Si: Fever, ileus, watery vaginal discharge, increasing creatinine

Crs: Requires rx. Important to maintain high index of suspicion

Cmplc: If not diagnosed promptly may lead to (1) urinoma and require percutaneous drainage, (2) nonfunctioning or hydronephrotic kidney (Urol Clin North Am 1977;4:17), (3) ureteral stricture

Lab: BUN and creatinine, UA, c + s

Xray: IVP (detects injury 94% of cases) and retrograde pyelogram (Campbell's Urology 1998;4(1):881–905)

Rx: Varies with degree of injury and time since injury. With minor injury, may pass JJ stent. If ureteral defect is large, will require exploration and repair. With iatrogenic suture ligation, may attempt laparoscopic suture removal and placement of JJ stent. If absorbable suture used, JJ stent can be placed until suture is absorbed. If unable to perform primary reapproximation, may consider ileal ureteral substitution, transureteroureterostomy or autotransplantation

2.26 CIRCUMCAVAL (RETROCAVAL) URETER

Cause: Embryologic abnormality related to persistence of subcardinal vein. The right ureter deviates medially behind inferior vena cava to cross in front of it from a medial to lateral direction, to course distally to the bladder

Epidem: Incidence 1 in 1200 cadavers (J Urol 1951;65:212). Male-to-female ratio 2.8:1. Patients usually present in the 3rd or 4th decade of life (BJU 1976;48:183)

Pathophys: Two clinical types. Type I: More common; assoc with hydronephrosis, a fishhook-shaped deformity of ureter to the level of the obstruction. Type II: Ureter passes behind the inferior vena cava at a higher level, and there may or may not be ureteral kinking and hydronephrosis

Sx: Asx or may present with sx of obstruction: Flank pain, N/V

Si: Hydronephrosis on renal US

Xray: IVP: May not visualize the ureter beyond area of obstruction. Renal US may demonstrate hydronephrosis and dilated proximal ureter if obstruction present. Retrograde ureteropyelography demonstrates S-curve of the ureter usually at L3–L4 and the retrocaval ureteral segment, but requires cystoscopy (BJU 1976;48:183). CT may help establish dx and avoid a retrograde study (J Comput Assist Tomogr 1986;10:1078)

Rx: If obstruction present, surgical rx involves ureteral transection and reapproximation anterolateral to inferior vena cava

2.27 RENAL CYST

Cause: Simple renal cysts are not connected to any part of nephron, but may originate initially from a portion of nephron

Epidem: May present anytime soon after birth to old age. Incidence increases with age: 20% incidence by age 40 yr and 33% by age 60 yr (BJU 1981;54:12)

Pathophys: May be singular or multiple, unilateral or bilateral. Vary in size from <1 cm to >10 cm; the majority <2 cm (Clin Radiol 1983;150:207)

Sx: Usually asx, but occasionally may cause pain

Si: Abdominal mass, hematuria, HT

Crs: Requires no rx or follow-up if a simple renal cyst

Cmplc: May bleed, become infected, and cause HT or obstruction

DiffDx: Cystic RCC

Lab: Not routinely indicated, but UA c + s if infection is suspected

Xray: US criteria for a simple cyst include (1) absence of internal echoes; (2) sharply defined, thin, and distinct margins; (3) good transmission of sound waves through the cyst with acoustic enhancement behind the cyst; (4) spherical or ovoid shape (Goldman SM, Hartman DS. The simple renal cysts. In: Pollack HM, ed. Clinical Urography. Philadelphia: Saunders, 1990:1603). CT criteria for a simple cyst include: (1) sharp, thin, distinct smooth walls and margins; (2) spherical or ovoid shape; (3) homogeneous content: density of −10 to +20 Hounsfield units and no enhancement with intravenous contrast. The Bosniak classification of renal cysts is as follows. Type I: Single, benign, fulfill the sonographic or CT criteria for simple cysts. Type II: Benign cystic lesions that are minimally complicated, such as by septations, small calcifications, infection, or high density. Type III: More complicated lesions with xray features seen in malignancy (lesions with more extensive calcification). Type IV: Cystic malignant tumors (Radiology 1986;158:1)

Rx: Asx simple cysts do not require rx. If benign simple cyst causes pain, obstruction, or HT, may unroof the cyst, open percutaneously, aspirate the fluid, and possibly inject a sclerosing agent, perform a percutaneous resection and intrarenal marsupialization, or laparoscopically unroof the cyst either transperitoneally or retroperitoneally (J Urol 1992;148:1835; J Endourol 1990;4:61)

2.28 AUTOSOMAL DOMINANT POLYCYSTIC KIDNEY DISEASE

Cause: Two genes for autosomal dominant polycystic kidney disease have been identified. One is on the short arm of chromosome 16 (BMJ 1986;292:851), accounting for 90–95% of cases. The second is on chromosome 4 and accounts for 5% of the cases (Nature Genet 1993;5:539). 100% penetrance. Appears to be a result of tubular epithelial cell hyperplasia and other factors (Kidney Int 1987;32:187;)

Epidem: Accounts for 9–10% of pts in Europe and U.S. who receive chronic hemodialysis (Proc Eur Dial Transplant Assoc 1978;15:36). Incidence is 1 in 500–1000. Most identified at 30–50 yr of age, but may also be detected in newborns. Renal failure is seldom seen before age 40. Men have more renal involvement than women, manifesting HT and renal insufficiency earlier than women (Adv IM 1993;38:409)

Pathophys: Micro and macrocysts are derived from the entire nephron. Assoc abnls: Cysts of the liver, pancreas, spleen and lungs, aneurysms, the circle of Willis. Berry aneurysms are present in 10–40%. About 9% of pts will die because of a subarachnoid bleed (Stroke 1990;21:291; Pediatr Urol 1984;7:4; J Neurosurg 1983;58:48), colonic diverticula, and mitral valve prolapse

Si: Palpable enlarged kidneys, HT (60%) appears to be renin-mediated secondary to stretching of the intrarenal vessels around the cysts (Nejm 1993;329:332) (Kidney Int 1990;38:1177), proteinuria, microscopic and gross hematuria in 50% pts (Am J Kidney Dis 1992;20:140; Nephron 1988;49:177), portal HT from enlarged cysts is rare (Nejm 1958;259:904)

Sx: Flank pain, abdominal pain, and renal colic secondary to clots or stones

Cmplc: Incidence of RCC is no higher in pts with autosomal dominant polycystic kidney disease than in the general population

DiffDx: R/o other renal cystic disease (Ann IM 1978;88:176). Multiple renal cysts: Benign, common retention cysts. MCDK: Compatible with life if unilateral; most not hereditary; assoc with ureteral atresia; most common type of renal cystic disease; assoc with little to no renal function and typically involute over time; increased incidence of contralateral VUR

Juvenile nephronophthisis/medullary cystic disease (Clin Pediatr 1986;25:90; Birth Defects 1974;10:32): Both conditions similar anatomically and clinically but have different modes of transmission and clinical onset. Juvenile nephronophthisis usually autosomal recessive and manifests at age 6–20 yr; medullary cystic disease is autosomal dominant and presents after the third decade. Both assoc with polyuria and polydipsia in >80% cases (Clin Pediatr 1986;25:90; Dialog Pediatr Urol 1984;7:3) as a result of salt wasting. Renal failure occurs 5–10 yr after initial presentation. Anemia is present. Rx is supportive and transplantation

Lab: Follow BUN, creatinine, and serum electrolytes; anemia often present with renal failure. Urine am specific gravity usually <1.015. Proteinuria often present

Xray: Abdominal US: Renal cysts and cysts in the liver and pancreas may be noted. In absence of a family hx of autosomal dominant polycystic kidney disease, a presumptive dx may be made if bilateral renal cysts identified and 2 or more of the following also present: bilateral renal enlargement; ≥3 hepatic cysts; cerebral artery aneurysm; a solitary cyst of arachnoid, pineal gland, pancreas, or spleen (Adv IM 1993;38:409). IVP: May look similar to autosomal recessive polycystic kidney disease. In adults, IVP usually demonstrates bilateral renal enlargement, calyceal distortion, and a "Swiss cheese" appearance in the nephrogram phase. CT may help detect cysts in other organs

Rx: Thorough family history. Monitor BP and follow renal function. Treat HT if present. Supportive rx of renal failure. If upper tract infection, use lipid-soluble abx, such as fluoroquinolones or Tm/S. Cyst pain may be treated with unroofing of cysts with relief of pain in 80% at 1 yr and 62% at 2 yr (J Am Soc Nephrol 1992;2:1219). Cyst aspiration alone is associated with increased risk of recurrence

2.29 AUTOSOMAL RECESSIVE POLYCYSTIC KIDNEY DISEASE

Cause: Inherited in autosomal recessive manner. Abnl of chromosome 6 (Prenat Diagn 1988;8:215; Am J Hum Genet 1995;56:110)

Epidem: Often diagnosed in the neonate, however may not become manifest until adolescence or young adulthood. Affects 1 in 5000–40,000 live births (Prenat Diagn 1988;8:215; Pediatr Kidney Dis 1992;2:1139)

Pathophys: Cysts derived primarily from collecting ducts. The earlier the age at which the dx is made, the more severe the disease. Often assoc with oligohydramnios and pulmonary hypoplasia

Crs: As many as 50% of affected newborns die within the first hours to days of life. Of those that survive the neonatal period, 50% are alive at 10 yr of age (J Pediatr 1989;115:867). All have varying degrees of congenital hepatic fibrosis

DiffDx: Autosomal dominant polycystic kidney disease, sporadic glomerulocystic kidney disease, renal vein thrombosis

Lab: BUN and creatinine may be normal at birth, but rise postnatally. Infants with disease evident at birth usually die within 2 mo as a result of uremia or respiratory distress. ABG

Xray: Renal US demonstrates enlarged, homogeneously hyperechogenic kidneys. IVP limited by renal function, but may see a characteristic radial or medullary streaking (sunburst) pattern, which is the dilated collecting tubules filled with contrast

Rx: Obtain a detailed family hx. No cure, initial rx is supportive. Those who survive the neonatal period will require rx for HT, CHF, and renal and hepatic failure. In many pts may consider hemodialysis and renal transplantation

2.30 ACQUIRED RENAL CYSTIC DISEASE

Cause: Appears to be a feature of end-stage renal disease, rather than response to dialysis. Cystic changes may be due to tubular obstruction secondary to interstitial fibrosis, deposition of calcium oxalate, proliferation of renal tubular epithelium, renal ischemia, or altered compliance of tubular basement membrane (Am J

Kidney Dis 1990;15:55; Virchows Arch Path Anat 1980;386:189; Kidney Int 1974;5:411). Some think decreased clearance of mitogenic polyamines and increased production of renal growth factors in pts on hemodialysis and peritoneal dialysis may lead to cyst formation (Am J Nephrol 1983;3:310; Lancet 1979;1:412)

Epidem: Regression of cysts after transplantation; if transplant fails and dialysis resumes, cysts return (Am J Nephrol 1983;3:310). Incidence 34–79% in pts on hemodialysis and appears to increase with duration on dialysis (Nejm 1984;310:390; Clin Nephrol 1980;14:1). Cysts also noted in pts undergoing long-standing peritoneal dialysis and those with chronic renal insufficiency not on dialysis (Nephron 1989;53:157; Am J Kidney Dis 1987;10:41; Lancet 1984;2:1482). Male:female 2.9:1 (Arch Pathol Lab Med 1986;110:592). May occur in children. Incidence higher in pts with end-stage renal disease secondary to nephrosclerosis (Semin Urol 1989;7:228)

Pathophys: Cysts occur primarily in the cortex, but may occur in the medulla. Usually affects both kidneys. Cysts derived from proximal tubular epithelium that retains secretory function (Nephrol Dial Transplant 1992;7:61307). Cysts may be lined by simple cuboidal, simple columnar, or hyperplastic multilayered epithelium with papillary projections (Urology 1981;17:260). Renal adenomas may arise from walls of the hyperplastic cysts; unclear whether these adenomas undergo malignant degeneration

Sx: Flank pain

Si: Hematuria, which may be secondary to rupture of an usupported sclerotic vessel in cyst wall (Urology 1981;17:260). If infected, cyst may cause a fever, elevated wbc

Cmplc: RCC: Incidence 20–25% (Am J Kidney Dis 1984;3:403). Incidence of RCC in these patients usually 3–6 × higher than in general population, and in blacks may be as much as 10 times higher (Med 1990;69:217). Infected cyst

Rx: Recommended that pts on hemodialysis for >3 yr duration undergo screening with US and/or CT. Frequency of screening is controversial and varies with presence/absence of cysts and size of solid masses. Risk of developing RCC in the native kidneys does not appear to decrease following renal transplantation and d/c dialysis

2.31 RENOVASCULAR HYPERTENSION

Nejm 1972;287:550

Cause: Atherosclerosis of renal arteries, renal artery fibromuscular hyperplasia, coarctation of aorta, other intrinsic renal disease

Epidem: 0.2–4% of all hypertensives (Can Med Assoc J 1973;117:492)

Pathophys: Decreased flow to renal juxtaglomerular apparatus causes renin production leading to angiotensin II (8-peptide), which causes arterial constriction, which increases aldosterone

Sx: None usually unless HT severe; then HA, CHF sx, epistaxis

Si: Coarctation lacks coincident radial and femoral pulses, rarely need to check temporal and radial in proximal type (Nejm 1973;288:899). Hemorrhages and exudates in fundi; 30% of patients with them have renovascular HT (Nejm 1979;301:1273). Abdominal bruit present in 60% (40% false neg), but 28% of all hypertensives have, so specif ≤35% (65% false pos) (Nejm 1967;276:1175); others find higher specif (90%), and if restricted to continuous bruits, sens 40%, specif 99% (Jama 1995;274:1299)

Cmplc: Like essential HT

Lab: (Ann IM 1992;117:845): Chem: Peripheral plasma renin (50–80% sens, 85% specif) with coincident urine Na^+ (Mod Concepts Cardiovasc Dis 1979;48:49) most useful if low since can then stop w/u; or renin levels before and after po captropril challenge show an increase to above 12 μgm/L/h; if creatinine <1.5 mg%, sens ≥75%, specif ≥90%. Uric acid elevated (Ann IM 1980;93:817). Hypokalemia; urinary K^+ <60 mEq/24 h after 3 d of 4+ gm Na^+ diet (G. Aagaard, 1969)

Xray: Renal scan before and after captopril 50 mg po shows decreased flow in affected kidney, 90% sens/specif (Ann IM 1992;117:845; Jama 1992;268:3353). Duplex US if hard to control HT and azotemia and/or peripheral vascular disease, 98% sens/specif (Ann IM 1995;122:883)

Rx: Percutaneous transluminal angioplasty (Nejm 1997;336:459; 1983;309:274). Surgical correction even if diminished renal function may help both BP and function (Nejm 1998;311:1070). In coarctation, pretreat with propranolol to prevent postop HT (Nejm 1985;312:1224)

3 Diseases of the Bladder

3.1 BACTERIAL CYSTITIS

Cause: Bacterial infection of lower urinary tract; uncomplicated UTI is a UTI in setting of functionally and structurally normal urinary tract. Complicated UTI: Pyelonephritis and/or structural or functional abnormality that decreases efficacy of abx rx

Epidem: Women > men except in neonatal period; prevalence in young women 30 × more than men; of recurrent UTI, 71–73% caused by reinfection of different organisms, rather than recurrence with same organism (Postgrad Med 1972;48:69)

Pathophys: Most bacteria enter urinary tract from fecal reservoir via ascent from urethra into bladder; occasionally may have seeding of kidney secondary to bacteremia; *E. coli* accts for 85% community acquired and 50% hospital acquired UTI. Factors affecting bacterial virulence and adherence and colonization include (1) hemolytic strains, (2) strains producing K ag (envelope or capsular polysaccharide ag), (3) pili (particularly type 1 pili and P pili) and fimbria, (4) alterations in number of vaginal epithelial and urethral receptor sites for *E. coli* (J Urol 1977;117:472). Increased risk with catheters, instrumentation, increased PVR

Sx: Dysuria, frequency, urgency

Si: Urge incontinence, hematuria

Crs: 50–80% of bacteriuric women untreated or treated with placebo will clear infection spontaneously (Postgrad Med 1972;48:69). Catheter-induced UTI has 2–4 × the mortality of non-catheter-induced UTI (Nejm 1982;307:637) and 1/3 resolve after removal without treatment; 90% will with single dose or 10-d rx (Ann IM 1991;114:713)

Cmplc: R/o vaginitis, herpes, pyelonephritis, VUR in children, IC, prostatitis, STD, bladder cancer, bladder instability

Lab:

Bact: c + s of midstream urine >10^5 organisms, >10^5 organisms in only 50% of truly infected women with sx; 10^2 a better criterion when symptomatic (Ann IM 1993;119:454; Nejm 1982;307:463).

Urine: UA shows pyuria, >5–6 wbc/hpf (10% false (−), 50% false (+) when have sx (Nejm 1982;307:463); hematuria; dipstick nitrite tests have high false-pos rates, so culture much better (Ped Infect Dis J 1991;10:651)

Xray: Unnecessary in most pts with GU infections, including most females with recurrent UTI, except pedi pts who should have VCUG and US with first UTI. May be indicated if suspecting obstruction, if UTI fails to resolve with appropriate abx, unusual organisms such as TB, fungus, or urea-splitting orgs

Rx: (Med Lett 1981;23:69) Tailor therapy to c + s results. Frequently used abx incl Tm/S, nitrofurantoin, fluoroquinolone, amoxicillin. Uncomplicated UTI treat for 3 d; 7 d for females with sx lasting >7 d, recent UTI, age >65 yr, DM, or pregnancy. Complicated UTI treat for 10–21 d (Eur Urol 1987;13(suppl 1):26; Ann IM 1987;106:467). Single-dose regimens cheaper, more convenient, but failure and recurrence rates higher (Arch IM 1992;152:1233; Ann IM 1988;108:350). Young males with no identifiable complicating factors treated with 7 d Tm/S, trimethoprim or a fluoroquinolone. Older males with UTI treat as if complicated UTI. Females with recurrent UTI may use prophylaxis with Tm/S 1/2 of single strength (40/200) tab qd (Nejm 1974;291:597) or postintercourse; is cost-effective if >3 UTIs/yr. Bladder anesthetics: phenazopyridine (Pyridium) 100–200 mg po tid for 2 d; stains urine dark orange. Future therapies: vaccines

3.2 EMPHYSEMATOUS CYSTITIS

Cause: Cmplc of UTI resulting in gas formation in bladder wall or lumen

Epidem: *E. coli* most common organism (Urol Int 1994;52:176; Ann Emerg Med 1990;19:404). Other organisms: *Proteus mirabilis, Nocardia, Candida, Enterobacter, Klebsiella, Streptococcus,*

Clostridium perfringens (J Urol 1992;147:134; Ann Emerg Med 1990;19:404; Am J Radiol 1961;86:850), rarely anaerobic organisms. Risk factors: urinary retention, chronic UTIs, DM, glycosuria (Urology 1985;25:88; Am J Radiol 1961;86:850). Females > males

Pathophys: High tissue glucose level along with impaired tissue and vascular response may provide setting for emphysematous infection (Urol Int 1994;52:176). Mechanism of gas formation: fermentation of glucose to CO_2 by gas-producing organisms in bladder (Br J Pathol 1995;49:334; BJU 1985;57:585). Assoc with intravesical fistula, diverticulitis, Crohn's disease, carcinoma of rectum/sigmoid (Ann Emerg Med 1990;19:404)

Sx: Frequency, urgency, nocturia, dysuria, suprapubic tenderness

Si: Pneumaturia

Lab: Urine c + s pos; UA, pyuria and hematuria

Xray:

 KUB: Thin radiolucent streaks or gas bubbles outlining bladder wall; air within bladder lumen with air fluid level in erect position

 CT: Gas within bladder wall or lumen; may reveal other intra-abdominal processes such as diverticulitis

 Cystoscopy: Gas bubbles within a shaggy erythematous bladder wall (J Urol 1943;49:808)

Rx: Abx, bladder drainage, control blood sugar. Prognosis usually good (Scand J Urol Nephrol 1997;31:309)

3.3 CANDIDA URINARY TRACT INFECTIONS

Cause: Fungal infection of the urinary tract. *C. albicans* most common (51%), *C. tropicalis* (25%), *C. parapsilosis* (12%), *Torulopsis glabrata* (9%), other species (3%) (Rev Infect Dis 1989;11:379)

Epidem: Increasing number of candida UTIs reported, partly as a result of increased use of broad-spectrum abx. Persistent candiduria in a critically ill surgical pt may portend disseminated infection with a mortality of 50% (J Trauma 1993;35:290)

Pathophys: DM, abx administration, steroid therapy, urine flow turbulence, congenital urinary tract anomalies, neurogenic bladder, indwelling catheters, and ileal conduits are risk factors for candidal infection (Rev Infect Dis 1982;4:1107). May involve vagina, bladder, genitalia, kidneys, ureters, prostate, epididymis

Sx: Dysuria, flank pain, nausea

Si: Urinary frequency, stranguria, pyuria, hematuria, pneumaturia, vomiting, oliguria, anuria

Lab: Urine microscopic: Candidal fungi with budding forms or pseudohyphae. Urinary casts containing fungi diagnostic of renal infection. Urine culture is pos if >10,000 on uncath or single-cath specimen. Blood cultures pos in pts with renal involvement (J Urol 1978;119:184). PCR rapidly and accurately identifies *Candida*; up to 100% sens and specif (J Urol 1996;156:154). No standardized serologic studies that can id upper tract involvement or invasive infections (Rev Infect Dis 1982;4:1107)

Xray: Renal US may identify fungal material in the collecting system, particularly in pediatric pts (Eur Urol 1985;11:188; Am J Radiol 1988;150:1331). CT displays the fungal accretions as a mass lesion with less attenuation than a stone

Rx: Removal of indwelling catheters or IV lines, improvement in nutritional parameters, d/c broad-spectrum abx. Candida cystitis: Bladder irritation with amphotericin B (50 mg amphotericin B in 1000 mL of water or D5W administered at 42 mL/h (1 L/d) successful in 80–92% of pts (Clin Infect Dis 1994;18:313; J Urol 1982;128:82). Localized renal pelvic and collecting sx infections: Percutaneous nephrostomy placement with irrigation with dose schedules similar to those used in bladder. May also percutaneously remove some fungal material from renal pelvis. Low-dose amphotericin B (10–24 mg/d for up to 15 d) used for infants with localized upper tract disease. If infection persists, then systemic rx indicated (J Urol 1988;140:338). Systemic rx for localized infection: Fluconazole (100 mg po bid for 10 d) is as effective as amphotericin B irrigations (91.4% vs 94.2%, $p = 0.322$) in rx of bladder infections (J Urol 1995;153:422A). Iv liposomal amphotericin 321–821 mg for 7–17 d helpful

Systemic rx for invasive or disseminated disease: Gold standard is IV amphotericin; dose varies; 6 mg/kg body weight used for critically ill surgical pts (Ann Surg 1982;195:177). Triazoles (fluconazole and itraconazole) also can be used. Comparison between iv amphotericin B (0.5–0.6 mg/kg body wt/d) and fluconazole (400 mg/d) in rx of candidemia in non-neutropenic pts demonstrates similar success (79% vs 70%, $p = 0.22$) (Nejm 1994;331:1325)

3.4 TUBERCULOSIS OF BLADDER, URETHRA

Cause: *Mycobacterium tuberculosis*; virtually always secondary to renal TB

Epidem: Usually starts at or around one or both ureteral orifices

Pathophys: Typically starts as inflammation around one or both ureteral orifices; bullous granulations may develop making visualization of the ureteral orifices difficult. If disease continues, may spread into muscle and eventually fibrose

Sx: Dysuria

Si: Urgency, frequency

Cmplc: Fibrosis may lead to UVJ obstruction or VUR. If extensive bladder involvement, may lead to small-capacity bladder. Rarely, extensive disease may lead to fistula formation into rectum

DiffDx: UTI, bladder cancer

Lab: Same as for renal TB

Rx: Chemotherapy as for renal TB. Surgical rx for UVJ obstruction may be indicated. In select cases, with small fibrosed bladders, bladder augmentation may be necessary. Cystectomy and creation of a neobladder may also be performed (J Urol 1998;159:202)

3.5 SCHISTOSOMIASIS

Cause: Digenetic (2 stages of multiplication: sexual in mature form and asexual in larval stage) parasitic trematode, *Schistosoma haematobium*

Epidem: 180 million people at risk for urinary schistosomiasis; 10–40 million will have obstructive uropathy or other sequelae (Bull WHO 1987;65:513; Pediatr Radiol 1986;16:225). Transmission occurs throughout African continent and Far and Middle East. Free-swimming cercaria penetrate skin or ingested, become schistosomula in blood, and mature into adults in blood vessels. Oviposition occurs primarily in pelvic lower urinary tract (Am J Trop Med Hyg 1977;26:696, 702)

Pathophys: 5 clinical stages:

1. Swimmer's itch: Cercarial penetration. Si/sx start 3–18 h after exposure, pruritic, macular rash at site of penetration

2. Acute schistosomiasis: 3–9 wk after infection, may be delayed for 4 mo; kata yama fever, onset of oviposition
3. Active schistosomiasis: Eggs deposited in tissues, traverse bladder or rectum and excreted in urine and feces; may be associated with hematuria and terminal dysuria
4. Chronic active: After some years, egg deposition and excretion occurs at a lower magnitude and sx less noticeable. Silent obstructive uropathy may develop related to fibrosis of bladder and ureters; may develop nephrotic syndrome caused by immune complex deposition in renal glomerulus
5. Chronic inactive: Viable eggs no longer detected in urine or tissue; of pts with obstructive uropathy, 40–60% present during inactive stage of their disease (Hum Pathol 1986;17:333)

Cmplc: Obstructive uropathy, urolithiasis, renal failure, bilharzial bladder cancer syndrome. Bilharzial bladder cancer typically presents at age 40–50 yr with squamous cell carcinoma of bladder (60–90%) and adenocarcinoma (5–15%) (Trans R Soc Trop Med Hyg 1990;84:551; BJU 1987;59:59; Trans R Soc Trop Med Hyg 1986;80:1009)

Lab: Terminally spined eggs in urine sediment diagnostic of active infection. Midday urine most likely to contain eggs (Tex Rpt Biol Med 1956;44:440). Rectal bx may show egg. Ziehl–Neelson stain. Hem: Increased eosinophils. Immunologic tests: Species-specific serine protease inhibitor (serpin) and its abs, detection of antigenemia or antigenuria by using circulating anodic antigen (CAA) and/or circulating cathodic antigen (CCA) dxs active disease and quantitates infection intensity (Parasitology 1994;108:519; Clin Infect Dis 1994;18:408; Am J Trop Med Hyg 1992;47:463). Intensity of infection correlates with number eggs per 10 mL/urine (Ann Soc Belg Med Trop 1988;68:123; Trop Med Parasitol 1986;37:223). Urine protein excretion parallels egg excretion and peaks at noon (Kid Int 1985;27:667), erythrocyte excretion delayed for about 6 h

Xray: KUB: May demonstrate calcifications within urinary tract; calcified bladder; also calcification of seminal vesicles, prostate, prostatic urethra, distal ureters. IVP: May see hydroureter, hydronephrosis, nonfunctioning kidney, ureteral stenosis, bladder/ureteral filling defects. VCUG identifies VUR, which occurs in 25% of infected ureters (Urology 1975;6:118). CT demonstrates obstructive uropathy and calcific lesions in urinary tract and colon (Br J Radiol 1990;63:357)

Rx: Metrifonate (Bilharcil) rx of choice in endemic areas. Dose: 7.5–10 mg/kg body wt, 3 doses at intervals of 14 d. Praziquantel (Biltricide) preferred drug in office practice. Single oral dose of 40 mg/kg. Other agents include hycanthone mesylate (Estrenal), niridazole (Ambilhar), and oltipraz. F/u at 3-mo intervals for 1 yr to assure cure or decrease in egg excretion. Surgical rx indicated for obstructive uropathy, stones, bladder cancer

3.6 HEMORRHAGIC CYSTITIS (HC)

Cause: In children may be secondary to adenovirus type 11 and 21 (Am J Dis Child 1973;26:605–608). Immunocompromised pts and pts undergoing BMT may be secondary to BK virus (a polyoma virus). Other causes: Acrolein, the urotoxic metabolite of cyclophosphamide and ifosfamide, XRT to the pelvis and bladder and an allergic reaction. May be secondary to medications including penicillin, NSAIDs, allopurinol, danazol, risperidone (J Urol 1998;160:159; BJU 1997;79:3; J Urol 1990;143:1)

Epidem: HC related to acrolein occurs in 4–40% of pts, mortality rate up to 75% (J Urol 1989;141:1063). 5–11.5% of pts rx with pelvic XRT have bladder cmplc, incl HC (J Urol 1993;150:332; S Afr Med J 1986;70:727)

Crs: Variable. Ranges from self-limiting to life-threatening hemorrhage

Cmplc: Secondary bladder cancer with cyclophosphamide therapy and pelvic XRT

DiffDx: R/o bacterial UTI, malignancy

Rx: Acrolein-related HC-aggressive hydration, frequent voiding, MESNA, CBI (J Urol 1995;153:637) help decrease incidence. Rx varies with etiology and severity of disease. That secondary to XRT and cyclophosphamide may be treated with (1) CBI; (2) intravesical alum, silver nitrate, carboprost tromethamine and formalin; (3) systemic therapy with episolom aminocaproic acid and sodium pentosapolysulphate; (4) electrocauterization; (5) neodymium:yag laser; (6) hydrostatic dilation; (7) urinary diversion; (8) hypogastric artery embolization (J Urol 1999;161:1747; 1997;154:2301; Lancet 1995;346:803; J Urol

1993;150:332; 1990;143:1). Hyperbaric oxygen has been used for XRT-induced HC (J Urol 1998;160:731) and may help prevent acrolein-related HC (J Urol 1998;159:1044)

3.7 INTERSTITIAL CYSTITIS (IC)

Cause: Exact cause unknown. Proposed etiologies include infections (Nejm 1994;331:1212), bladder mastocytosis and mast cell activation (Urol Clin North Am 1994;21:41), defect in epithelial permeability barrier of bladder surface glycosaminoglycans (GAG) (J Urol 1993;150:845), urine abnormalities that may be toxic (Urol Clin North Am 1994;21:153), alterations in sensory nervous system (Neuroscience 1992;48:187), and autoimmune-related causes (Eur Urol 1980;6:10)

Epidem: Rare in childhood. Median age of onset is 40 yr. Occurs more often in females (female:male ratio 9:1). 100% increased incidence in Jewish people (Neurourol Urodynam 1990;9:241). Up to 50% of affected people experience spontaneous remissions, probably unrelated to rx, that last for 1 to 80 mo (AUA Update Series 1999;2:10). Assoc diseases incl allergies, allergic symptoms, fibromyalgia, vulvodynia, migraine headaches, endometriosis, chronic fatigue syndrome, incontinence, asthma, systemic lupus erythematosis, inflammatory bowel disease, and Sjögren's syndrome (Urology 1997;49:52; Urol Clin North Am 1994;21:20; J Musculoskel Pain 1993;1:295)

Pathophys: No pathognomonic histopathologic features of IC. Histopathology used to r/o other possible diseases, such as carcinoma, eosinophilic cystitis, and TB cystitis. Hunner's ulcers visible during hydrodistention in 20% of affected patients (Urol Clin North Am 1994;21:20). Refer to NIADDK Research definition of IC (Table 3–1)

Sx: Pain in lower abdomen, perineum, low back, or vagina; 75% of patients note exacerbation of sx with intercourse

Si: Severe urinary frequency and urgency, voiding at least 8 times d, tender bladder base during pelvic examination, nocturia

Crs: No sure cure for interstitial cystitis. Severity and frequency of sx vary

Cmplc: May have significant adverse affect on quality of life

Table 3–1. NIADDK Research Definition of Interstitial Cystitis

Required Criteria
- Glomerulations or Hunner's ulcers on cytoscopic examination
- Pain associated with bladder or urinary urgency
- Cystoscopy & hydrodistention: Glomerulations in ≥3 quadrants of bladder and ≥10 per quadrant; bladder distended under anesthesia to 80–100 cm H_2O for 1–2 min 1–2 times for evaluation of glomerulations

Exclusion Criteria
- Bladder capacity >350 mL on awake cystometry
- Absence of intense urge to void at 150 mL H_2O during cystometry (fill rate 30–100 mL/min)
- Presence of phasic involuntary bladder contractions during cystometry
- Duration of symptoms <9 mo
- No nocturia
- Symptomatic relief with abx, anticholinergics, antispasmodics, urinary antiseptics
- Awake daytime frequency <8 times/d
- Dx of bacterial cystitis or prostatitis within 3 mo
- Bladder or lower ureteral calculi
- Active genital herpes
- Uterine, cervical, vaginal, or urethral cancer
- Urethral diverticulum
- Chemical (cyclophosphamide), tuberculous or radiation cystitis
- Benign or malignant bladder tumors
- Vaginitis
- Age <18 yr

NIADDK-National Institute of Arthritis, Diabetes, Digestive and Kidney Diseases.

DiffDx: Other forms of cystitis, DI, bladder cancer, voiding dysfunction

Lab: UA, c + s, urine cytology

Xray: Not routinely indicated

Other Eval: Urodynamic evaluation helpful to assess bladder capacity and rule out DI. Cystoscopy under anesthesia with hydrodistention of the bladder and bladder bxs can be performed to look for glomerulations and Hunner's ulcers and to assess bladder capacity. Hydrodistention is also therapeutic

Rx: Initial therapeutic approach is hydrodistention of bladder under anesthesia, which is diagnostic and therapeutic

Medical Therapy: Amitryptyline: success rates of 64–90% at a follow-up of 2–14 mo. Start at 25 mg qhs and increase to 75 mg qhs over 2 wk. Most valuable in patients with significant pain (Urol Clin North Am 1994;21:63; J Urol 1990;143:279).

Hydroxyzine: 25 mg po qhs to start; increase to 50 mg at night and 25 mg in morning. Improves symptoms in 40–55% of pts (Urol 1997;49:108). Pentosan polysulfate (Elmiron): A GAG-layer replenishing agent. Administered as 100 mg po tid. Symptoms improve in 6–32% of pts (J Urol 1993;150:845; Urol 1988;51:381). Other oral agents have been tried: nifedipine, nalmefene, antispasmodics, L-arginine, misoprostol

Intravesical Therapy: DMSO is primary intravesical therapy for IC (Urol Clin North Am 1994;21:73; Urology 1987;29:17); may be used alone or in comb with steroids, heparin, bicarbonate. Rx varies from 1–2 instillations per wk for 4–8 wk. Objective response in 93% of cases and subjective response in 53% (J Urol 1998;159:1483). Chlorpactin WCS 90: A 0.4% solution is administered under anesthesia. Average success rate 72% with an average 6-mo duration of response. Contraindicated if VUR is present (Urology 1979;13:389). Other possible intravesical agents include capsaicin, silver nitrate, lidocaine, doxorubicin, hyaluronic acid, BCG, cromolyn sodium

Other Therapies: Nerve stimulation: Transcutaneous electric nerve stimulation has shown good results in 20% of nonulcer IC patients (Urol Clin North Am 1994;21:131). Surgical rx used as a last resort. Supravesical diversion with cystectomy is rarely used in patients for whom all other therapies have failed

3.8 EOSINOPHILIC CYSTITIS

Urology 1995;46:729

Cause: Allergic cystitis

Epidem: Increased risk in pts with history of allergies, including food and environmental allergies, parasitic infections (J Urol 1982;127:132; J Peds 1968;73:340), intravesical agents such as mitomycin and thiotepa (BJU 1987;59:547). Other risk factors: bronchial asthma, atopic diseases. Associated conditions: Glanzmann's thombasthenia and eosinophilic gastroenteritis. In children, males > females; the reverse in adults (Urology 1995;46:729)

Pathophys: ? Exposure to foreign protein substance, which acts as antigenic stimulus in bladder. IgE-mediated release of eosinophilic chemotactic factor and release of lysosomal enzymes (J Urol 1982;127:132)

Sx: Urgency, dysuria, suprapubic tenderness

Si: Hematuria

Cmplc: Bladder wall fibrosis leading to decreased compliance and bladder capacity; if severe, may lead to hydronephrosis

DiffDx: Invasive bladder carcinoma (Scand J Urol Nephrol 1993;27:275–77)

Lab: UA may show pyuria, microhematuria, and occasionally eosinophilia. Serum: Eosinophilia may be seen. Cystoscopy: Erythematous, velvety, raised lesions in bladder or edematous bladder mucosa with ulcers

Xray: VCUG may demonstrate VUR, bladder wall thickening, and small bladder capacity. Bladder bx: Eosinophilic infiltrate scattered throughout lamina propria and muscularis (Arch Pathol Lab Med 1984;108:728)

Rx: Some cases self-limiting. If persistent or recurrent, treat with oral abx, antihistamines, steroids (J Urol 1982;127:132). NSAIDs also useful (J Urol 1990;144:1464). Allergy evaluation and removal of potential allergens

---

3.9 COLOVESICAL FISTULA

Cause: Underlying bowel disease

Epidem: Most commonly associated with diverticulitis (50%) (Surg Gynecol Obstet 1991;173:91). Crohn's disease, cancer of the colon, or other pelvic malignancies may also cause fistula formation

Pathophys: Communication between bowel and bladder. Spontaneous closure unusual. Fistula on left side of dome of bladder is likely to be result of diverticular disease; that on right side is likely to be associated with Crohn's disease

Sx/Si: Urinary frequency and urgency, dysuria, pneumaturia, suprapubic discomfort, gastrointestinal symptoms

Lab: Urine c + s may demonstrate multiple bacterial species present

Xray: CT helps identify fistula—may see gas in bladder or fistula tract. Cystoscopy and cystogram useful in identifying location of fistula (Surg Gynecol Obstet 1991;173:91)

Rx: Rx based on underlying bowel disease and often involves removal of affected bowel segment and bladder closure

3.10 INVERTED PAPILLOMA

Cause: Unknown. Benign, may be result of chronic inflammation or BOO (J Urol 1997;158:1500)

Epidem: Most common in trigone and bladder neck; may occur in prostatic urethra and ureter (J Urol 1990;143:802). Male:female ratio 3:1–7:1 (Pathology 1994;15:279), 6% multicentric (Cancer 1978;42:708), 50–79 yr of age (J Urol 1997;158:1500)

Pathophys: Histopathology: papillary fronds project into fibrovascular stroma of bladder with thin layer of urothelium overlying lesion. May contain cystitis cystica (see 3.13) or squamous metaplasia (see 3.11). If high immunoreactivity for p53 may be susceptible to malignant transformation (BJU 1996;77:55)

Sx: Flank pain, lower urinary tract symptoms

Si: Hematuria

Crs: Rare cases of malignant transformation (Cancer 1978;42:1984). May be associated with coexistent TCC of bladder (see 3.14) or hx of previously treated TCC. Rare recurrence

DiffDx: Bladder neoplasm

Lab: Urine cytology to r/o malignant cells

Xray: IVP may show filling defect, obstruction, or may be normal

Cystoscopy: Lesion typically appears as small raised nodule

Rx: TUR of bladder lesion

3.11 SQUAMOUS METAPLASIA OF BLADDER

Cause: Proliferative lesion

Epidem: Most common in bladder neck and trigone. In other areas of bladder, may be precancerous (J Urol 1954;71:718); females > males

Pathophys: In the absence of cellular atypia or marked keratinization is probably benign; in females, involvement of trigone is normal

variant, occurring under hormonal influence (J Urol
   1979;122:317; Am J Anat 1962;111:319)
Lab: Cystoscopy and bladder bx if lesion appears suspicious
Rx: Not necessary

3.12 NEPHROGENIC ADENOMA

Cause: Metaplastic response of urothelium to trauma, infection or XRT.
   87% assoc with surgery, trauma, infection, calculi (Urology
   1987;29:237)
Epidem: Typically males. Any age, long time after insult (J Urol
   1989;142:1545)
Pathophys: Histopathol: Resembles primitive renal tubules (J Urol
   1999;161:605). Bladder most common (84%) (Urol Int
   1994;53:227), even augmented bladders and ileal conduits
   (J Urol 1996;155:1410; 1987;137:491)
Sx: Dysuria, urinary frequency
Si: Lesions vary from small to >7 cm (J Urol 1999;161:605); hematuria
Crs: Benign lesion. May occur with IC (Urology 1985;26:498)
DiffDx: Mesonephric adenocarcinoma, TCC, cystitis
Lab: Urine cytology to r/o malignant cells
Cystoscopy: May appear similar to muscle invasive TCC (J Urol
   1999;161:605) or be papillary and exophytic (BJU 1999;84:169)
Rx: TUR lesion. Radical cystectomy if malignant lesion identified

3.13 CYSTITIS GLANDULARIS

Cause: Benign, may be premalignant, proliferative disorder of mucus-
   producing glands in submucosa and mucosa of bladder (Urology
   1998;51:112)
Epidem: Incidence 0.1–1.9% (J Urol 1971;105:671; 1968;100:462).
   Associated with chronic UTIs, obstruction, stones. Other possible
   etiologies: avitaminosis, toxic metabolites, hormonal imbalance,
   carcinogen-related (Proc Roy Soc Med 1970;63:239), humoral
   immunology alterations (Br J Surg 1972;59:69). Increased

incidence in those with pelvic lipomatosis (J Urol 1993;110:397; Urology 1975;5:383). Occurs in children (Urology 1990;36:364)

Pathophys: May evolve from Brunn's epithelial nests in setting of chronic infection or irritation or may be congenital reflecting partial origin of bladder from embryonic cloaca (Hum Pathol 1997;28:1152)

Sx: Dysuria, urgency, frequency

Cmplc: Adenocarcinoma of bladder assoc with cystitis glandularis. May evolve into adenocarcinoma (J Urol 1991;145:364;1972;108:568)

Si: Hematuria, voiding mucus

DiffDx: Von Brunn's nests: Normal urothelium in lamina propria found in 89% of normal bladders at autopsy (J Urol 1979;122:317). Cystitis cystica: Similar to Von Brunn's nests, but urothelium has undergone liquefaction, present in 60% of normal bladders at autopsy (J Urol 1979;122:317). Cystitis follicularis: Submucosal lymphoid follicles non-neoplastic response to chronic bacterial infection

Lab: Urine c + s ± pos, UA ± pyuria. Cystoscopy: Often multiple, lobulated or papillary lesions

Rx: TUR to establish dx. Treat inciting disease process. 1-yr f/up cysto recommended given increased incidence of coexistant adenocarcinoma (Urology 1998;51:112)

3.14 BLADDER CANCER

Cause: Neoplasm. TCC accounts for 90% of bladder cancers. Less commonly identified malignancies include squamous cell carcinoma, adenocarcinoma, urachal carcinoma, and nonurothelial bladder tumors such as carcinosarcoma, spindle cell carcinoma, sarcoma, leiomyosarcoma, rhabdomyosarcoma, neurofibroma, pheochromocytoma, lymphoma, and mets

Epidem: Most common site of cancer in urinary tract. Male:female ratio 3:1. Fourth most common cancer in males and fifth most common cancer in females. Incidence of bladder cancer appears to be increasing (Hematol Oncol Clin North Am 1992;6:1), but incidence of advanced bladder cancer and mortality rates from bladder cancer are decreasing (Annual Cancer Stat Rev 1987. Bethesda: U.S. Dept. HHS, NIH Publ. 92-2789)

Pathophys: Risk factors: cigarette smoking, occupational chemical exposures (aniline dye workers), dietary, analgesic abuse, chronic infection, schistosomiasis infection, pelvic XRT, and cytotoxic agents (cyclophosphamide). Loss of chromosome 9q is seen more frequently with superficial bladder cancers; loss of 17q, 5q and 3p is more commonly associated with invasive bladder cancer (J Urol 1992;148:44). Bladder cancer also associated with genetic alterations that affect cell growth and proliferation, such as tumor suppressor gene p53 (possibly found on chromosome 17p) and overexpression of retinoblastoma gene (Rb)

Squamous Cell Carcinoma: Associated with chronic infection with *Schistosoma haematobium*. Other causes include chronic irritation from urinary calculi, long-term indwelling Foley catheters, chronic UTI, or bladder diverticula

Adenocarcinoma: Most common type of cancer in exstrophic bladders. Develops in response to chronic inflammation and irritation (J Urol 1984;131:262;1983;130:1180)

Urachal Carcinoma: Develops outside the bladder and invades into the bladder wall beneath normal epithelium (J Urol 1954;71:715)

Prognostic Factors: Tumor type, tumor grade, and stage

DiffDx: Cystitis cystica, inverted papilloma, nephrogenic adenoma, squamous metaplasia, pseudosarcoma, condyloma accuminata, UTI

Sx: 1/3 patients with bladder cancer will have irritative voiding symptoms: urgency, frequency, and dysuria. Flank pain may accompany ureteral obstruction. Bone pain may be secondary to bony mets

Si: Hematuria: Gross or microscopic, if lesion is large may have a palpable mass on rectal or bimanual examination, hydronephrosis if assoc with ureteral obstruction. With advanced disease may have weight loss and lower extremity edema

Lab: UA, c + s to r/o UTI and check for hematuria. Urine cytology: More sensitive in pts with high-grade tumors or CIS. False-neg rate up to 20%. False-pos cytology in 1–12% (Diagn Cytopathol 1989;5:117). Serum alkaline phosphatase if lesion is invasive

Xray: Upper tract evaluation with an IVP to r/o upper tract tumors: 10% chance (Urol Clin North Am 1992;19:455). Chest xray to r/o lung mets. CT of abdomen/pelvis in pts with muscle-invasive disease. Bone scan indicated if alkaline phosphatase elevated

Other Tests: Cystoscopy to identify lesion(s)

Rx: Cystoscopy and TUR of lesion(s) for pathologic evaluation and staging. If unresectable, then deep bxs. Rx based on type of cancer, stage of the cancer, and patient's overall medical condition

TNM Bladder Cancer Classification

- T0   No evidence of primary tumor
- Ta   Noninvasive papillary carcinoma
- Tis   Carcinoma in situ
- T1   Tumor invades subepithelial connective tissue
- T2   Tumor invades muscle
- T2a   Superficial muscle
- T2b   Deep muscle
- T3   Tumor invades perivesical tissue
- T3a   Microscopically
- T3b   Macroscopically
- T4   Tumor invades adjacent organs/pelvic structures

(American Joint Committee on Cancer Staging. Hermanek P, Sobin LH, eds. UICC—International Union Against Cancer TNM Classification of Malignant Tumors, 4th ed. Heidelberg: Springer-Verlag, 1987:135)

Squamous Cell Carcinoma: Aggressive surgical rx if possible: Radical cystectomy, BPLND ± urethrectomy (J Urol 1980;123:850)

Adenocarcinoma: Radical cystectomy and BPLND best chance for cure. Responds poorly to XRT and chemotherapy (J Urol 1989;141:17; Cancer 1989;64:2448)

Urachal Carcinoma: Rx of choice is radical cystectomy with an en bloc excision of the urachus. XRT and chemotherapy have not been very effective

Transitional-Cell Carcinoma: Rx based on grade and stage of the tumor

   CIS: Assoc with increased risk of invasive disease. Most effective rx is intravesical BCG. It produces complete remission in 50–65% of pts. Other intravesical agents include mitomycin C, doxorubicin, interferon, valrubisin, and thiotepa. Pts should be followed with regular cystoscopies and urine cytologies

   Ta: Adjuvant intravesical rx indicated for high risk of recurrence: high-grade tumors, multiple tumors, hx recurrent tumors, persistence of CIS (J Urol 1988;139:283). Follow with regular cystoscopies and cytologies

   T1: Consider reresection if any question of residual tumor. Approximately 30% will progress to a higher stage tumor, particularly high-grade tumors. Consider intravesical rx with high-grade tumors. Routine cystoscopy and urine cytologies

T2–T4 N0–N2: Best treated with radical cystectomy, BPLND, and urinary diversion or orthotopic bladder. In select cases, may consider bladder preservation (chemotherapy plus XRT), TUR, or partial cystectomy

Metastatic TCCA: Chemotherapy with MVAC: methotrexate, vinblastine, adriamycin, and cisplatin

Palliative Therapy: XRT for painful bony mets; for bladder bleeding consider intravesical 1% alum (J Urol 1982;128:929), 1–10% formalin (make sure no reflux) (Br J Urol 1970;42:738), or hypogastric artery embolization for severe bleeding. Palliative cystectomy and urinary diversion for patients with severe bladder symptoms

Prognosis: For noninvasive TCC bladder treated with TUR there is a 70% 5-yr survival rate (J Urol 1992;148:1413). 10–15% of these pts will require more aggressive rx. Nearly all pts with mets die within 2 yr (J Clin Oncol 1992;10:1066; Urology 1980;16:142). 10–35% of pts with limited regional nodal involvement survive 5 yr after radical cystectomy and BPLND. 18–35% of pts with T2, T3a disease will eventually die from their cancer

3.15 BLADDER CALCULI

Cause: Dietary in children in such areas as Thailand, Indonesia, North Africa, and the Middle and Near East (Fogarty Int Center Proc 1977;37). BOO and UTI in adults

Epidem: Uric acid stones are identified in about 50% of pts with bladder stones (Urology 1991;37:240). Calcium phosphate stones are also noted. Usually a single stone, but may be multiple, especially when bladder diverticulum is present. Pediatric bladder calculi in endemic areas are ammonium acid urate and/or calcium oxalate

Pathophys: Dietary, concentrated acid urine, and outlet obstruction. Pediatric stones related to low phosphate, high oxalate, and high acid diet (J Urol 1988;140:461; BJU 1976;48:617; Am J Clin Nutr 1974;27:877)

Sx: Intermittent painful urination; severe pain may occur at the end of urination as stone impacts at the bladder neck

Si: Terminal hematuria, interrupted urine stream related to obstruction from the stone

Crs: Size may continue to increase over time

Cmplc: Urinary retention, recurrent UTI

Lab: UA, c + s

Xray: Filling defect in bladder on IVP. May be detected on bladder US. If stone is calcium containing, may be identified on plain film of the abdomen and pelvis

Other Studies: Cystoscopy confirms presence of a stone or stones

Rx: Endoscopic or open stone removal, depending on stone size. Relief of obstruction, correction of bladder stasis, and removal of foreign bodies decrease risk of recurrence. Pts with chronic indwelling catheters who are at increased risk for stone formation may use an irrigation of 0.25–0.5% acetic acid solution 2–3 times/d

3.16 BLADDER TRAUMA

Cause: Blunt or penetrating trauma to lower abdomen/pelvis

Epidem: In civilian populations blunt trauma accounts for 67–86% of bladder rupture and penetrating trauma for 14–33% (J Urol 1984;132:254; Urol Clin North Am 1982;9:243). 90% of bladder ruptures from blunt trauma due to motor vehicle accidents. Pelvic fractures identified in 89–100% of extraperitoneal bladder ruptures

Pathophys: Type of bladder rupture related to bladder volume. Empty bladder more susceptible to extraperitoneal bladder rupture; full bladder prone to intraperitoneal rupture via a blowout at the dome. Increased risk of intraperitoneal rupture with excess alcohol intake. 10% of patients have combined intraperitoneal and extraperitoneal bladder rupture

Sx: Diffuse lower abdominal tenderness, suprapubic pain

Si: Hematuria, suprapubic and pelvic ecchymosis, anuria

Crs: Once identified, requires rx. High index of suspicion if pelvic fracture present

Cmplc: Urinary extravasation, extensive pelvic and abdominal wall abscess and necrosis, peritonitis, and intra-abdominal abscess

Lab: UA, c + s if patient is able to void, CBC, electrolytes, BUN, creatinine

Xray: Cystogram if suspect bladder rupture. Bladder should be filled with at least 300 mL of water-soluble iodinated contrast with AP, oblique or lateral, and postdrainage films. If associated penetrating trauma, CT may be indicated

Rx: Bladder wall contusion if no evidence of extravasation on cystogram, Foley catheter drainage indicated for a few days until hematuria clears and patient is ambulatory. Intraperitoneal rupture best treated with surgical exploration and repair. Extraperitoneal rupture may heal with urethral catheter drainage for 7–10 d in absence of penetrating trauma

3.17 VESICOVAGINAL FISTULA

Cause: In developed countries, most common cause is iatrogenic damage to bladder during surgery. Gynecologic surgery accounts for 70–80%, with majority occurring after abdominal hysterectomy. Far less common causes include erosion into bladder from a pessary or vaginal diaphragm, erosion from an intravesical foreign body, or tuberculosis of the bladder (Am J Obstet Gynecol 1990;163:589; BJU 1988;62:271; Aust NZ J Obstet Gynecol 1984;24:225). In undeveloped countries, vesicovaginal fistulas are obstetric related

Pathophys: In undeveloped countries in which women have children at a young age, prolonged difficult labor may lead to excessive pressure on the bladder and bladder necrosis. Many gynecologic procedure-related vesicovaginal fistulas develop from unsuspected bladder injury, which leads to urinary extravasation and urinoma formation, which then drains into the vaginal cuff (Surg Gyncecol Obstet 1988;166:409). XRT-related fistulas may develop mo to yr after XRT

Sx: Excessive abdominal pain, distention, or paralytic ileus, sx of bladder instability

Si: Hematuria, painless watery discharge from vagina. Volume of leakage varies depending on size and location of fistula

Crs: Postoperative fistulas usually become manifest 3–14 d postoperatively

Lab: UA, c + s; BUN and creatinine of the vaginal fluid; if BUN and creatinine values exceed that of serum (usually 20×), urinary leakage is confirmed

Cystoscopy: To identify number, size, and location of the fistulas and to assess the degree of bladder inflammation. May instill fluid via the cystoscope and examine vagina with speculum for leakage. If XRT-related, assess bladder capacity and bx fistula to r/o cancer

Xray: Cystogram may identify the vesicovaginal fistula; IVP or retrograde studies should be performed on pts with vesicovaginal fistulas to r/o an associated ureterovaginal fistula (10–25% incidence) (Urol Clin North Am 1985;12:361; J Urol 1980;123:370)

Dye Studies: Instill methylene blue or indigo carmine into bladder and examine vagina; may also insert tampon into vagina after bladder filled; staining at top of tampon consistent with vesicovaginal fistula

Rx: Timing of surgery based on degree of bladder inflammation. XRT-induced fistulas: Wait until the acute radiation injury subsides; at least 6–12 mo after XRT. Small fistulas (<2–3 mm) may be fulgurated and catheter placed for 2–4 wk. 71% success rate (J Urol 1994;152:1443;1980;123:367). Large fistulas require transvaginal or transabdominal repair, depending on surgeon's experience. Contraindications to vaginal approach: Narrow vagina, high-vault fistula, and close proximity to ureteral orifice. Vaginal repair success rate 85–95% (J Urol 1990;144:34; Am J Obstet Gynecol 1971;4:524), less for XRT-induced fistulas, which also require additional procedures like interposition of vascular pedicle. Transabdominal approach useful for complex fistulas, those close to ureteral orifice, interposition of flaps, and if simultaneous bladder surgery indicated. Success rates 86–100% (Int Urol Nephrol 1985;17:159; J Urol 1989;141:513). Cmplcs of surgery: Recurrence of fistula, ileus, stress incontinence, infection, ureteral injury, bleeding, bladder stones, rectal injury, small capacity of bladder. With a transvaginal approach other risks include narrowing of the upper vagina and dyspareunia

3.18 CYSTOCELE

Cause: Descent of anterior vaginal wall and overlying bladder base due to either overstretching and attenuation of anterior vaginal wall or due to detachment or elongation of anterolateral vaginal supports to pelvic diaphragm

Epidem: 70–80% of all cystoceles caused by damage to lateral support (Am J Obstet Gynecol 1976;126:568)

Pathophys:

Cystocele grading by physical examination:

Grade 1 Minimal bladder descent

Grade 2 Descent to the introitus with stress maneuver

Grade 3 Descent to the introitus at rest

Grade 4 Descent beyond the introitus

Cystocele grading on fluoroscopy:

Grade 1 Descent of the bladder base just below the symphysis

Grade 2 Descent 2–5 cm below the symphysis

Grade 3 Descent >5 cm below the symphysis

(Campbell's Urology, 1998;7(32):1075)

Sx: Small cystoceles often asx. Large cystoceles may cause dyspareunia, back pain

Si: Vaginal bulge, UTI, increased PVR, renal insufficiency

DiffDx: Enterocele, rectocele, uterine prolapse

Lab: UA, c + s r/o UTI

Xray: Bladder scan PVR to ensure adequate bladder emptying. Renal US should be obtained with grade 4 cystocele to r/o silent hydronephrosis

Urodynamics helpful to assess hypermobility of urethra, demonstrate stress incontinence, document PVR, and help grade the severity of the cystocele defect (Adv Urol 1992;5:121)

Rx: Three primary types of cystocele repair: Transabdominal procedures (effective for small cystoceles), Kelly plication/anterior colporrhaphy and its modifications, and transvaginal suspension procedures. Cmplc of cystocele repair: De novo urge incontinence (14%), de novo stress incontinence (2%), recurrent cystocele. Urinary retention, ureteral obstruction, inadvertent cystotomy, and significant bleeding are rare (Urol Clin North Am 1995;22:641; J Urol 1991;146:988)

3.19 URODYNAMIC TESTING

Several components incl uroflowmetry, PVR determination, CMG, and a VCUG. Fluoroscopy used to evaluate bladder and urethral configuration, to determine when leakage occurs, and to detect VUR. Urethral pressure measurement and/or sphincter EMG may be added in select cases. Urodynamics helpful in assessing pts with neurogenic bladder, urinary incontinence, outflow obstruction, or voiding dysfunction of unclear etiology

Uroflow: Volume of urine voided per urethra per unit of time (mL/sec), reflects combined activity of bladder muscle (detrusor) and urethra. Parameters to assess include (1) maximum flow rate (normal for males >60 yr >13 mL/sec; females >50 yr >18 mL/sec) (Urol Clin North Am 1979;6:71), (2) total volume of urine voided, (3) urine flow pattern

CMG and VCUG: CMG is continuous measurement of bladder pressure during filling. Used to determine bladder compliance (change in volume/change in pressure) (Scand J Urol Suppl 1998;114:5) and to identify presence of uninhibited bladder contractions (phasic increases in detrusor pressure). Presence of uninhibited contractions is called DI in absence of neurologic lesion and DH in presence of neurologic abnormality. VCUG is fluoroscopic visualization of the bladder and urethra during filling and voiding and is often used to detect VUR, bladder diverticuli, and posterior urethral valves

Pressure Flow Study: Simultaneous measurement of bladder pressure and urine flow rate throughout voiding cycle. Useful to evaluate possible BOO

Videourodynamics: CMG plus pressure flow study and EMG if indicated are performed with simultaneous fluoroscopic imaging of the lower urinary tract. Leak point pressures obtained during urodynamic study to assess risk of upper urinary tract damage (bladder leak point pressure; BLPP) and the integrity of the intrinsic sphincter (Valsalva leak point pressure; VLPP)

BLPP: Often obtained in individuals with neurogenic bladder, particularly children, is bladder pressure at which urethral leakage occurs. BLPP >40 cm H_2O associated with risk of upper tract damage (J Urol 1981;126:205)

VLPP: Pressure that abdominal musculature must generate to overcome resistance of sphincteric mechanism for leakage to occur. A normal sphincter will not leak, no matter how high VLPP. VLPP >90 cm H_2O is seen in pts with anatomic stress incontinence; VLPP <60 cm H_2O indicates intrinsic sphincter deficiency

EMG: Used to assess for detrusor–sphincter dyssynergia (DSD); measures sphincteric activity during filling and voiding; normally increase in pelvic muscle activity during filling and cessation during detrusor contraction and voiding. Failure of relaxation of pelvic muscles or increased contraction during voiding suggests DSD

3.20 INCONTINENCE

Cause: May be transient (reversible) or established (persistent). Etiologies of transient incontinence include DIAPPERS: delirium, infection, atrophic urethritis/vaginitis, pharmacologic, psychologic, endocrine, restricted mobility, and stool-fecal impaction. Persistent incontinence may be due to a disorder of the bladder, bladder outlet, or both, including urge incontinence, stress incontinence, functional incontinence, and mixed incontinence (Postgrad Med 1991;90:99)

Epidem: In the community, 5–15% of the elderly suffer from incontinence at least weekly and >50% in a nursing home setting (BMJ 1981;282:940; Aging 1979;8:81; Gerontol Clin 1969;11:330)

Pathophys: Pharmacologic causes: Meds that promote incontinence include sedative hypnotics, diuretics, anticholinergics, adrenergic agents, and calcium channel blockers (Med Grand Rounds 1984;3:281). Endocrine causes of polyuria such as hypercalcemia and hyperglycemia may lead to incontinence

URGE INCONTINENCE

Cause: Incontinence associated with an active detrusor contraction. At least 1/3 of elderly pts will have coexistent impaired detrusor contractility (Jama 1987;257:3076)

Lab: CMG demonstrates phasic increases in bladder pressure assoc with involuntary loss of urine

Rx: Anticholinergic agents in pts with adequate contractility (Lancet 1995;346:94):

Propantheline 15–30 mg po q4–6 h

Oxybutynin (Ditropan), also a muscle relaxant, 2.5–5 mg po bid to qid

Ditropan XL 5–15+ mg/d

Detrol (tolterodine) 1–2 mg po qd to bid

Imipramine HCL (Tofranil): An alpha agonist and anticholinergic; 10 mg po tid.

Side effects of anticholinergics: dry mouth, blurry vision, flushing, tachycardia, constipation, drowsiness. Ditropan XL has less dry mouth side effects. If impaired contractility plus instability, may require CIC in addition to anticholinergic. Other therapies: Kegel exercises, biofeedback

OVERFLOW INCONTINENCE

Cause: BOO (BPH, bladder neck obstruction, urethral stricture or atonic bladder)

Sx: Decreased force of stream, urinary frequency, feeling of incomplete emptying, lower abdominal distention, incontinence without urgency

Lab: Large PVR on bladder scan or catheterization. 100% of nl males have residual volumes <12 mL (J Urol 1963;96:180). PVR increases with age. If large PVR, check serum BUN and creatinine to r/o renal insufficiency

Rx: CIC at intervals to keep PVRs consistently <500 cc. Evaluate for possible obstructing lesions and rx if bladder function is adequate. Urodynamic studies may help determine etiology of increased PVR and assess detrusor function

Med that increase bladder contractility: Bethanechol (Urocholine), a cholinergic agent, 20–100 mg tid to qid; increases bladder pressure but results with bladder emptying are poor. Side effects include flushing, N/V, diarrhea, GI cramps, bronchospasm, HA, salivation, sweating, and visual changes

Meds that decrease outlet resistance (work on bladder neck and urethra): Doxazosin (Cardura), terazosin (Hytrin), tamsulosin (Flomax)

Striated muscle relaxants, work on external urethral sphincter: Diazepam (Valium), 10–15 mg po qid; dantrolene (Dantrium), 25–100 mg qd to qid; baclofen (Lioresal): 20 mg qid, indicated for skeletal muscle spasticity

STRESS INCONTINENCE

Cause: Abnormal urethral closure function, loss of normal function of supporting structures of the urethra from anatomic, hormonal or neurologic causes

Type 0 Complaint of stress incontinence without clinical demonstration of leakage

Type 1 Demonstrable leakage in response to stress, but little descent of bladder neck and urethra

Type 2 Incontinence in response to stress with >2.0 cm descent of bladder neck and urethra

Type 3 Bladder neck and urethra are open at rest without a bladder contraction due to intrinsic urethral damage ⌣ denervation of the urethra (Urol Clin North Am 1991;18:197)

Type 1 and 2 associated with Valsalva leak point pressures >60 and ranging up to 120–130 cm H_2O. With type 3, Valsalva leak point pressures are as low as 5 and as high as 30–40 cm H_2O (J Urol 1993;150:1452)

Pathophys: Type 1&2: Bladder neck and proximal urethra function as the continence zone (Urol Clin North Am 1985;12:207) and pressure in this area is higher than intravesical pressure, except during voiding. With adequate support, increased abdominal pressure is evenly distributed to bladder and continence zone. With loss of pelvic support, there is descent of bladder and proximal urethra, creating unequal distribution of abdominal pressure, with more going to the bladder and less to the continence zone, thus allowing bladder pressures to exceed those of the continence zone, leading to leakage. Type 3: Sphincteric incontinence may be due to prior surgery, atrophic urethritis, neurologic problems, and in males RRPX and TURP

Rx: Weight reduction, pelvic floor muscle (Kegel) exercises, estrogen therapy for low-risk postmenopausal females, medical rx, and surgical rx (bladder neck suspension, pubovaginal sling, collagen injection) (J Am Ger Soc 1983;31:476). Alpha-adrenergic agents: pseudoephedrine 30–60 mg po qid, imipramine HCl (Tofranil) 10 mg po tid

3.21 HEMATURIA

Def: Presence of >3 rbcs/hpf; may be microscopic or gross.

Urine dipstick vs. UA: Pos dipstick indicates hematuria, hemoglobinuria, or myoglobinuria. Sens of dipstick >90%, specif lower secondary to higher false-pos rate with dipstick (Jama 1985;253:1956).

False-pos dipstick may be secondary to contamination with menstrual blood; dehydration, which increases urine specific gravity, which leads to increased concentration of erythrocytes and hgb; exercise; ingestion of large amounts of ascorbic acid (vitamin C), which inhibits peroxidase reactions; ingestion of vitamins and food products with high concentration of oxidants

DiffDx: Gross hematuria: Hematuria, hemoglobinuria, myoglobinuria, anthocyanin (in beets and blackberries), chronic lead and mercury poisoning, phenolphthalein, phenothiazines, and rifampin

Work up hematuria to r/o medical renal disease, stones, infections, tumors. 20% of asx males >50 yr with (+) dipsitck have urologic pathology; 5–15% have bladder cancer (J Urol 1987;137:919)

Renal (medical) vs urologic disease: Casts, significant protein, and dysmorphic red cells suggest medical renal disease

Lab: Evaluation for urologic disease: UA to confirm hematuria and r/o significant proteinuria, urine c + s to r/o UTI, serum BUN and creatinine, IVP to assess upper urinary tracts, urine cytology to r/o presence of malignant cells, cystoscopy to assess bladder

4 Diseases of the Urethra

4.1 REITER'S SYNDROME

Bull Rheum Dis 1987;37:1; Ann IM 1984;100:207; Nejm
  1983;309:1606

Cause: Autoimmune

Epidem: Systemic illness assoc with preceding urethritis due to gc or
  Chlamydia; or enteritis due to *Yersinea, Salmonella, Shigella,*
  Campylobacter, Neisseria, or *Ureaplasma* (Bull Rheum Dis
  1990;39:1)

Sx: 2–4 wk incubation period (urethritis or enteritis). First urethritis
  (85%), cervicitis and/or prostatitis; then red eye (conjunctivitis);
  then wks later, arthritis, arthralgias (99%), especially peripheral
  and lower extremities, especially heels, ankles, knees, low back

Si: Peripheral arthritis and purulent urethral discharge (95%); red eye
  from conjunctivitis (40%) or uveitis (8%); fever (37%); painless
  skin or mucous membrane lesions (32%), especially circinate
  balanitis and keratodermia blennorrhagia (looks like pustular
  psoriasis)

Crs: 80% resolve after 4–12 mo; 20% chronic

Cmplc: Aortitis (1%); heart block (1%)

DiffDx: R/o chronic lyme arthritis, gc, erythema multiforme, Behçet's
  syndrome, psoriasis, ankylosing spondylitis

Lab:

  Joint Fluid: wbc 5000–50,000, mostly polys but lower % than
    gc with more monos, occasionally with ingested polys
    (LE phenomenon) (Ann IM 1967;66:677).

  Serol: RA titer (–), HLA B 27 (+) in 60–75%, but only 8% of people
    with (+) titer have Reiter's (Ann IM 1982;96:70)

Xray: Periosteal new bone formation along shafts (phalanges)

Rx: Tetracycline therapy for presumed chlamydia of pt and partner
  (Bull Rheum Dis 1992;40:1), NSAIDs

4.2 GONORRHEA (GC)

Cause: *Neisseria gonorrhoeae*

Epidem: Venereal. Common in teenagers and racial and ethnic minorities. Risk increases as number of sexual contacts with infected partners increase. Coincident infection in 15% male heterosexuals, 25% females (Nejm 1984;310:545)

Pathophys: Infects mucous membranes of GU tract (Nejm 1985;312:1683)

Sx:

Male: Urethral discharge, usually profuse and purulent, but up to 2/3 asx (Nejm1974;290:117)

Female: Bartholin cyst (80% acute Bartholin's gland cyst infections are due to gc); vaginal discharge, dysuria, pelvic inflammatory disease, pain typically occurring with menses or pregnancy, abnormal menstrual bleeding due to endometriosis

Si: Urethral discharge. In female, abdominal distention, "Chandelier sign" (severe pain with cervical motion), pus in cervix

Crs: Incubation period 3–10 d

DiffDx: *Trichomonas, Candida, Chlamydia* (Nejm 1974;291:1175), syphilis, Reiter's syndrome, appendicitis in female

Lab:

Bact: Gram stain, in male 1st, culture only if unclear on Gram stain; in female, smear of cleanly wiped cervix to look for >3 polys/hpf with intracellular gram-neg cocci, has 67% sens, 98% specif. If hx of oral genital contact, pharyngeal specimen, in homosexual male and all women rectal swab

Culture: In male only if unclear on smear. In female, Gram stain more difficult to interpret and less sensitive than smears from male urethra, thus culture on selective media still often necessary (J Clin Path 1998;51:564). Reculture all after rx and recheck VDRL if neg first time. Penicillinase-producing strains now in U.S.

Rx: CDC recommendations for rx of gonococcal urethritis: Ceftriaxone 125 mg im, 1st choice for uncomplicated gc infections of pharynx, anorectum, cervix, and urethra. Also treat for possible coexisting chlamydia (MMWR 1989;38:1)

DISEASES OF THE URETHRA

4.3 NONGONOCOCCAL URETHRITIS (NGU)

Cause: *Chlamydia trachomatis* accounts for 30–50% of cases; 20–50% men with NGU may have *Ureaplasma urealyticum*

Epidem: Incidence 2.5 times that of gc urethritis (Epidemiol Rev 1983;5:96)

Pathophys: Smoking may be a risk factor (Sex Transm Dis 1988;15:119) as well as being circumcised (Am J Public Health 1987;77:452)

Crs: Incubation period usually 1 to 5 wk

Sx: Dysuria, urethral discharge

Lab: Gram stain urethral swab: >4 polys/hpf suggestive of urethritis. Endourethral swab rather than urethral exudates or urine, place 2–4 mm inside urethra; preliminary culture available in 2–3 d. Direct fluorescent ab (DFA): Rapidly detects *C. trachomatis* elementary bodies; enzyme immunoassay (EIA) can also be used, pos test color changes when viewed with spectrophotometer, results in 24 h; PCR: Highly specif test for fluorescence of chlamydial nucleic acids; contamination by foreign DNA a problem (Gen Clin Pathol 1991;44:1)

Rx: CDC recommendations: Tetracycline 500 mg qid for 7 d or doxycycline 100 mg po bid or erythromycin 500 mg po qid for 7 d; rx partners. Single 1-gm dose of azithromycin found to be therapeutically equivalent to tetracyclines and may improve compliance. If recurrent or persistent, r/o other causes of urethritis; if no cause found or *Ureaplasma urealyticum* present, erythromycin base 500 mg qid for 14 d (Urol Clin North Am 1984;11:55)

4.4 GENITAL ULCERS

Cause: A variety of organisms may cause genital ulcers incl herpes simplex virus, *Treponema pallidum*, *Haemophilus ducreyi*, *Chlamydia trachomatis*, and *Calymmatobacterium granulomatis*

Epidem: Herpes simplex is 10 times more common than gonorrhea and chlamydia in college students. Incidence of syphilis is higher than it has been in 30 yr, with many infections occurring in populations that have a high prevalence of HIV (Cutis 1993;52:72). Chancroid has increased in importance in the U.S. (Ann IM 1985;102:805) and is a risk factor in the acquisition of HIV in heterosexual intercourse (Scand J Infect Dis 1990;69:181; Nejm 1988;319:274). Granuloma inguinale is rare in the U.S. but is the major cause of genital ulcers in Southeast India, New Guinea, the Carribean, parts of South America, South Africa, and Australia

Pathophys: See Table 4–1

Sx: See Table 4–1

Si: See Table 4–1

Crs: See Table 4–1

Cmplc: Secondary infections, scarring

DiffDx: See Table 4–1

Rx: See Table 4–1

4.5 TUBERCULOSIS OF THE URETHRA

BJU 1973;45:432

Cause: *Mycobacterium tuberculosis*

Epidem: Very rare; occurs via spread from another area in genital tract

Pathophys: 2 phases: (1) acute (urethral discharge with involvement of epididymis, prostate, other parts of GU tract); and (2) chronic (urethral obstruction)

Sx: In chronic phase, obstructive voiding sx

Si: In acute phase, urethral discharge; in chronic phase: decreased force of stream

DiffDx: Sexually transmitted diseases, urethral stricture

Lab: Culture of urethral discharge for TB

Rx: Antituberculosis chemotherapy; if stricture present, internal urethrotomy

Table 4-1. Genital Ulcers

	Genital Herpes	Syphilis	Chancroid	Lymphogranuloma Venereum	Granuloma Inguinale
Cause	Herpes simplex virus, usually type II but 10–25% cases assoc with type I (Nejm 1981;305:315; J Antimicrob Chem 1983;12:79)	Spirochete, *Treponema pallidum* incubation about 3 wk	*Haemophilus ducreyi* gram (–) coccobacilli, "school of fish" appearance on Gram stain	*Chlamydia trachomatis* serotypes L1, L2, and L3	*Calymmatobacterium granulomatis* encapsulated gram (+) bacteria
SSX	1st episode more severe than recurrent, dysuria 44% males, 83% females, weakness, sensory loss, impotence, malaise, anorexia, urinary retention, constipation, fever, tender adenopathy	Primary: Painless lesion (chancre) heals in 3–4 wk, adenopathy. Papule becomes indurated and punched out. Secondary: Skin rash, painless adenopathy, low-grade fever malaise, pharyngitis, laryngitis, arthralgias. Tertiary: sx reflect organ, sx affected; classic neurologic sx include tabes dorsalis, Argyll–Roberts pupil	Incubation 1–4 d, nonindurated, ragged, undermined painful ulcer may be assoc with painful adenopathy. Base of ulcer is friable. If untreated becomes suppurated with periadenitis (bubo formation). Chronic draining sinuses may occur	Incubation 3–30 d. 3 stages: (1) small asx papule or herpetiform lesion; (2) occurs days to wks after 1st, tender, discrete lymphadenopathy with fever, myalgias, possible meningitis; (3) extensive periadenitis that spreads to surrounding tissues yielding inflammatory mass, abscesses within coalesce to form bubo that may rupture and cause fistula (Arch Pathol 1939;27:1032)	Incubation 8–80 d. Primary: Small painless papule or indurated nodule; lesion ulcerates, leads to beefy-red, granulomatous ulcer with rolled edges that bleed easily; lesions may coalesce; spontaneous healing with scar formation; may cause lymphedema and elephantiasis of external genitalia from obstruction of lymphatics

Lab	Viral isolation by culture most sensitive but takes 5 d; in situ DNA hybridization (J Infect Dis 1983;147:829)	Dark-field exam quickest and most direct for primary, secondary, tertiary. VDRL most often used to follow pt response to rx. RPR should be nonreactive in primary syphilis 1 yr after successful rx and 2 yr after successful rx of secondary syphilis (Jama 1985;253:1269). Fluorescent antibody absorbed test (FTA abs) once + remains so, T. pallidum hemagglutination assay (TPHA, MHA-TP) (Sex Transm Dis 1980;7:111)	Gram stain smear obtained from base of lesion shows gram (–) coccobacilli in chains or clusters (Derm Clin 1994;12:1). Definitive dx culture on specific media	Microimmunofluorescent ab test most specific and best. Bx of lesion shows heavy infiltration with neutrophils and plasma cells (Derm Clin 1994;12:1; Genitourin Med 1992;68:130)	Histologic exam of punch bx specimen taken from edge of active lesion or from scraping edge shows intracellular Donovan bodies on stained smear in direct immunofluorescent test
Rx	Acyclovir drug of choice, inhibits viral polymerase, acts as chain terminator. Primary: Oral acyclovir 200 mg 5 x/d for 7–10 d or 400 mg po tid For 7–10 d. Acyclovir decreases viral shedding, time to crusting, healing of lesions, duration of pain and itching in primary. Recurrent herpes: May decrease duration of viral shedding and time to crusting. If taken in prodromal period, may abort episode in some (J Am Acad Derm 1986;15:256) 400 mg po tid X 7–10 d. Prophylactic: 400 mg po bid decreases recurrences; safe, effective up to 5 yr (Arch Derm 1993;129:582). Consider for pts with >6–8 recurrences/yr	Benzathine penicillin G 2.4 million units im × 1 for primary. Pen allergic: Doxycycline 200 mg po bid × 15 d	Ceftriaxone 250 mg im × 1 (Rev Infect Dis 1990;12:S580) or azithromycin 1 gm po dose or erythromycin base 500 mg po qid for 7 d or Cipro 500 mg po bid for 3 d. HIV + patients don't respond as well	Doxycycline 100 mg po bid for 21 d or erythromycin base 500 mg po qid for 21 d. Local wound care	Rx continued until epithelialization occurs. Doxycycline 100 mg po bid × 3 wk min or erythromycin 500 mg po qid or Tm/S DS 1 tab po bid for min 3 wk. Optimum abx and rx duration not well defined

4.6 MALE URETHRAL CARCINOMA

Urol Clin North Am 1992;19:347

Cause: Neoplasm; appears to be related to chronic inflammation

Epidem: Rare, most commonly identified in men >50 yr. Incidence of urethral stricture in males with cancer of urethra 24–76%. Most frequent site of cancer is bulbomembranous urethra (60%), penile urethra (30%), and prostatic urethra (10%). Better prognosis with more distal lesions

Pathophys: Histologically, 80% are squamous cell carcinomas, 15% TCCs, 5% adenocarcinomas and undifferentiated tumors. The TNM classification of carcinoma of the urethra follows:

Primary Tumor (T) (Male and Female)

TX Primary tumor cannot be assessed

T0 No evidence of primary tumor

Ta Noninvasive papillary, polypoid, or verrucous carcinoma

Tis Carcinoma in situ

T1 Tumor invades subepithelial connective tissue

T2 Tumor invades corpus spongiosum, prostate, or periurethral muscle

T3 Tumor invades corpus cavernosum or beyond prostatic capsule, anterior vagina, or bladder neck

T4 Tumor invades other adjacent organs

Regional Lymph Nodes (N)

NX Regional lymph nodes cannot be assessed

N0 No regional lymph node mets

N1 Mets in single lymph node, ≤2 cm in greatest dimension

N2 Mets in single lymph node, >2 cm, <5 cm in greatest dimension; or multiple lymph nodes, none >5 cm in greatest dimension

N3 Mets in a lymph node >5 cm in greatest dimension

Distant Metastasis (M)

MX Presence of distant mets cannot be assessed

M0 No distant mets

M1 Distant mets

(Beahrs O, Henson D, Huller R, Kennedy BJ. Manual for Staging Cancer. Philadelphia: Lippincott, 1992)

Sx: Urinary frequency, penile pain, dysuria

Si: Palpable urethral mass, palpable inguinal nodes (20%), decreased force of stream, urethral bleeding, urethrocutaneous fistula

Lab: Urine c + s to r/o UTI. Cystoscopy and bx to confirm malignancy

Rx: Depends on location and extent of tumor. Cancer of distal urethra if superficial may be treated with TUR and fulguration. If invasive then partial or total penectomy indicated. Lymph node dissection indicated if palpable inguinal adenopathy. If cancer involves bulbomembranous urethra and is superficial, may be treated with TUR and fulguration or segmental excision and urethral reapproximation. If invasive, radical cystoprostatectomy indicated along with total penectomy and pelvic lymph node dissection. May require more extensive surgery. Prognosis poor with invasive disease. For cancer of prostatic urethra, may be TCC or adenocarcinoma. If lesion is superficial, TUR (J Urol 1989;141:853). If lesion is invasive, cystoprostatectomy and total urethrectomy. Five-year survival with invasive disease is <20%. XRT is used as palliative rx, as an adjunct to surgical rx and as primary rx (Cancer 1978;41:1313)

4.7 FEMALE URETHRAL CARCINOMA

Campbell's Urology 1998;7(108):3395–3409

Cause: May be related to chronic irritation, infection

Epidem: Affects women over age 50 more commonly and whites more frequently. Squamous cell carcinoma is most common (60%), followed by TCC (20%), adenocarcinoma (10%), undifferentiated carcinomas and sarcomas (8%), and melanoma (2%). Most are locally advanced at dx and involve proximal 1/3 or entire urethra. Primary TCC of female urethra does not appear to be a part of multifocal TCC disease (Cancer 1990;65:1237; Urology 1977;10:583)

Sx: Dysuria, urinary frequency

Si: Palpable urethral mass or induration, foul-smelling urethral discharge. Clinically palpable lymph nodes found in 1/3 of pts and represent cancer mets in 90%

DiffDx: Infected diverticulum, urethral caruncle, papilloma, adenoma, urethral polyp

Lab: Urine c + s to r/o UTI. Pelvic examination, cystourethroscopy and bx under anesthesia

Xray: Chest xray to rule out lung mets. CT of abdomen/pelvis to check for mets and lymph node involvement. If patient has bowel or bone sx then barium enema, bone scan

Rx: Rx depends on tumor location and extent. Local excision may be performed for superficial, localized distal tumors. With proximal invasive lesions, extensive surgery is often required, including total urethrectomy, cystectomy, lymph node dissection, and removal of most/all of vagina. Bladder-sparing surgery may be performed in select pts with locally advanced TCC of the urethra (J Urol 1993;150:1135). XRT successful for small distal lesions (67% survival vs 83% for surgery), but minimally effective for proximal tumors (20%) (Urol Clin North Am 1992;19:373). Other options incl combined therapies such as preoperative chemotherapy and XRT followed by radical cystourethrectomy

4.8 URETHRAL TRAUMA

Cause: Blunt or penetrating trauma to pelvis, perineum, or penis in males

Epidem: Males > females. Injury of posterior urethra in 5% males with pelvic fracture (J Urol 1983;130:712). Anterior urethral injury more common than posterior urethral injury. Anterior most often result of straddle injury or blunt trauma to perineum (Urol Clin North Am 1989;16:329). Pelvic fracture uncommon with anterior urethral injury

Pathophys: Strong shearing forces in high-speed blunt and crush injuries or high-velocity penetrating trauma can tear attachments of prostate and puboprostatic ligaments from the pelvic floor, leading to a tear in posterior urethra. In females with urethral trauma, severe pelvic fracture and bony displacement can lead to laceration of bladder neck and vagina.

Male urethral injuries classified as posterior (prostatic and membranous urethral injuries above or including the urogenital diaphragm) and anterior (injuries of bulbous and penile urethra). Classification of male posterior urethral injuries:

Type I   Stretching and elongation without rupture of the posterior urethra

Type II   Partial or complete disruption of prostatomembranous urethra

Type III Partial or complete disruption of prostatomembranous urethra and rupture of urogenital diaphragm and bulbous urethra (J Urol 1977;118:575)

Anterior urethral injuries: If rupture contained within Buck's fascia, urine and blood dissect along penile shaft. If rupture extends through Buck's fascia, then urine and blood may extravasate along attachments of Colles' fascia—butterfly configuration in perineum

Sx: Suprapubic pain

Si: Inability to void, blood at meatus, gross hematuria, perineal ecchymosis, high-riding prostate on DRE

Lab: Hgb/crit to r/o significant bleeding

Xray: Pelvic films to assess pelvic fractures. CT scan if intra-abdominal injury suspected. Retrograde urethrography indicated in pts with suspected urethral trauma; need AP and oblique films

Rx:

Treatment of Posterior Urethral Injury

Type I injury: Foley catheter for 3–5 d. Type II injury: If tear is partial, catheter may be advanced into bladder fluoroscopically or endoscopically and remains in place 7–14 d with VCUG obtained after removal. Type III and complete type II: Rx is controversial. Traditionally, open suprapubic tube placement performed initially with delayed repair (endoscopic or open) >3 mo postinjury when pelvic hematoma resolved. Primary repair recommended for severe prostatomembranous dislocation, major bladder neck laceration, and concomitant vascular or rectal injury (J Urol 1992;148:1428; J Trauma 1991;31:1390; Campbell's Urology 1992;6:2957–3032). Cmplc: Incontinence, impotence, urethral stricture

Treatment of Anterior Urethral Injury

Contusion: Foley catheter placement. Urethral disruption: Surgical exploration, debridement, and direct repair. Severe cases with extensive tissue loss: Initial urinary diversion may be indicated

4.9 URETHRAL DIVERTICULUM

Cause: May be congenital or acquired (secondary to infection, injury)

Epidem: In males, congenital diverticula may occur in prostatic urethra (a Müllerian duct remnant) in intersex disorders or represent an enlarged utricle in males with proximal hypospadias (J Urol 1980;123:407). Acquired may occur as cmplc of hypospadias repair. In females, may result from dilation of periurethral glands or may follow maternal birth trauma. Incidence in females is estimated at 1.4–4.7% (Am J Obstet Gynecol 1978;13:432; 1965;92:106)

Pathophys: In males, a congenital diverticulum may result from incomplete development of urethra. In females, obstruction of periurethral glands may lead to infection and microabscess formation with decompression into urethral lumen leading to diverticulum formation

Sx: Dysuria, urinary frequency, tenderness on palpation

Si: In males with posthypospadias repair diverticula, the diverticulum may be visible as an outpouching of urethra during voiding. Other signs: Recurrent UTIs, postvoid dribbling, outflow obstruction, tender urethral mass on vaginal examination in females. May note blood, pus, or urine from meatus with compression of anterior vaginal wall

Cmplc: Adenocarcinoma, infection, calculi

DiffDx: In females, cystocele, Gartner's duct cyst, vaginal inclusion cyst, urethral carcinoma, Skene's abscess, vaginal carcinoma, ectopic ureterocele

Lab: Urine c + s to r/o UTI. Cystoscopy may be able to localize the mouth of the diverticulum. VCUG useful to detect diverticula, particularly in females (Urology 1987;30:407). Positive pressure urethrography indicated in select cases (BJU 1981;53:353)

Rx: Congenital diverticuli in males may be asx and not require rx. If large and sx they may be excised transvesically or transsacrally (J Urol 1982;17:796). A postoperative diverticulum may be approached through the penis. In females, urethral diverticula are traditionally excised transvaginally (Atlas Urol Clin North Am 1994;2:73). In select cases, diverticulum may be marsupialized

5 Diseases of the Testes, Scrotum, and Intra-Scrotal Contents

5.1 EPIDIDYMITIS/EPIDIDYMO-ORCHITIS

Cause: Males <35, condition is usually caused by STDs (chlamydia, gonorrhea, ureaplasma). In older men, gram-negative bacteria more common. Coliforms are identified in homosexual men who practice anal intercourse (J Infect Dis 1987;155:134; J Urol 1979;12:750)

Epidem: Rare in people under age 18 yr; peak incidence is at age 32 yr

Pathophys: Inflammation localized to the epididymis or also involving testis

Sx: Usually gradual in onset and of under 6 wk duration

Si: Swollen, tender epididymis (+/–testis), possible scrotal wall erythema, nontender testis

Crs: Lasts 7–10 d if treated; improved with scrotal elevation, decreased activity

Cmplc: Abscess formation, testicular infarction, chronic pain, infertility

DiffDx: R/O testicular torsion (most common during adolescence, torsion often presents with more acute onset and often assoc with N/V, loss of cremasteric reflexes, and testicular pain)

Lab: UA, c + s

Xray: Scrotal US may be helpful if abscess or torsion suspected. Testicular torsion is a clinical diagnosis

Rx: Abx: Pt <40 yr, ceftriaxone 250 mg im × 1 or ciprofloxacin 500 mg po × 1, then doxycycline 100 mg po bid × 10 d. Pt >40 yr, broad-spectrum abx (Tm/S, quinolone) (Med Let 1995;37:117;1994;36:1; 1999;41:86), NSAID, decreased activity, scrotal elevation

5.2 GENITAL CONDYLOMA

Cause: Usually a STD: Human papillomavirus (HPV) type 6 or 11 typically. HPV types 1 and 2 can cause skin and genital warts

Epidem: Increasing in incidence worldwide. Warts may appear months to years after acquisition of HPV. Consistent condom use significantly decreases risk (Sex Transm Infect 1999;75:312). Previous chlamydial infection in both males and females is negatively associated with risk of genital warts. In males, risk factors incl younger age, cigarette smoking, alcohol consumption, and greater number of lifetime partners. In females, risk factors incl younger age, never having been married, unemployed, cigarette smoking, alcohol consumption (Sex Transm Infect 1999;75:312)

Pathophys: Natural hx marked by fluctuating course of visible lesions, latency, and recurrence. Some lesions regress, some persist, others appear after rx. Most clinically apparent lesions will resolve in mo to yr. Three types of lesions: cauliflower-like condyloma accuminata usually involve moist surfaces, keratotic and small popular warts are usually on dry surfaces, and subclinical "flat" warts are found on any mucosal or cutaneous surfaces

Sx: 1–6 mo incubation; may cause pain

Si: Clinical infections present as lesion

DiffDx: Penile cancer, molluscum contagiosum

Rx: CDC guidelines for condyloma: Rx of genital warts should be guided by preference of pt. Extensive rxs, toxic rxs, and procedures that result in scarring should be avoided. Goal of rx is removal of exophytic warts and amelioration of si/sx, not eradication of HPV (MMWR 1993;2:83). Rx options (Am J Med 1997;104:28) are as follows:

Cytotoxic rx: Eliminate genital warts by destroying affected tissue. (1) Trichloroacetic acid (TCA), causes chemical coagulation of condyloma; 80–90% solution applied directly to genital wart and repeated wkly if necessary; best on small, moist warts. Side effects: discomfort, ulcers, and scarring (Sex Transm Dis 1993;20:344). 36% pts develop new lesions in 2 mo (Genitourin Med 1987;63:390). Limit to area <10 cm². (2) Podophyllin, plant compound that causes tissue necrosis by arresting cells in mitosis; 10–25% podophyllin can be applied wkly for up to 6 wk for

1–4 h, then wash off. 50% respond, but warts recur in 40%. Side effects: local skin reaction including redness, tenderness, itching, burning pain, and swelling. Systemic side effects include bone marrow depression. Ineffective on relativity dry anogenital areas. (3) Podofilox (Condylox), the major biologically active ligand of podophyllum resin. Use 0.5% solution for topical application bid for 3 d, hold 4 d, and repeat 4–6 times as necessary. Limit to wart area ≤10 cm². Appears to be more effective and works faster than podophyllin (Genitourin Med 1988;64:263) but recurrences are common. 30% recurrence within 1 mo of rx (Obstet Gynecol 1991;77:735; Lancet 1989;1:831). Less successful for sessile warts or lesions on dry skin surfaces (Sex Transm Infect 1999;75:192). (4) 5-Fluorouracil (5 FU), inhibits cell growth by interfering with DNA and RNA synthesis; applied 1–3 times wk for up to 10 h; useful for meatal lesions; up to 75% clearance with recurrence <10% (J Reprod Med 1990;35:384; Obstet Gynecol 1984;64:773). Side effects include local irritation

Ablative rx: (1) Cryotherapy, liquid nitrogen employed for freezing and destruction of wart and small area of surrounding tissue. Effective in about 75% with recurrence in 21% (Int J Dermatol 1985;24:535). Can be painful. (2) Laser rx, popular choice for rx of lesions that have not responded to other rxs. Recurrence rates 6–17% to 49% (Obstet Gynecol 1984;64:773; 1980;55:711; 1982;59:105; 1984;63:703). (3) Electrosurgery, involves fulguration of tissue affected by genital warts. Loop electrosurgical excision involves electroexcision and fulguration. Requires local or general anesthesia depending on size of lesion. More effective than podophyllin or cryotherapy, but has a similar recurrence rate (Genitourin Med 1990;66:16). Side effects include bleeding, scarring, infection. (4) Surgical excision, yields 90% clearance rate and 20% recurrence rate (J Gynecol Surg 1995;11:41; Br J Surg 1989;76:1067). (5) Interferon-alpha, approved for intra-lesional rx of warts. Recombinant IFN-alpha₂ᵦ (Intron A) 3 injections/wk for 3 wk, natural IFN-alpha (Alferon N) 2 injections/wk for 8 wk. Clearance rates 36–53%, recurrence rates of 20–25% (Jama 1988;259:533; RCH Dermatol 1986;122:272; Nejm 1986;315:1059). Side effects: Flu-like sx, leukopenia, pain

Newer rx: (1) 5 FU/epinephrine, injectable gel shows complete response in 25–71% varying with size of lesion, 3-mo recurrence rate of 39% in pts with complete response (Am J Med

1997;102:28). (2) Solid formulation Podofilox, gel and cream forms appear to have response profiles similar to the solution, easier to use. (3) Imiquimod, immune-response modifier is potent inducer of IFN-alpha and enhances cell-mediated cytolytic activity against viral agents (Antiviral Res 1988;10:209); also induces a variety of cytokines (J Leukoc Biol 1995;58:365). Use of 5% cream yields clearance rates of 50%. Can be left on for 6–10 h and use 3 d wk for 16 wk (Jama 2000;283:175). Side effects include erythema, erosion, excoriation, and flaking. (4) Vaccine therapy: Both prophylactic and therapeutic vaccines are under investigation

5.3 MALE GENITAL TB (TB OF EPIDIDYMIS, TESTIS, AND PROSTATE)

Scand J Urol Nephrol 1993;27:425

Cause: *Mycobacterium tuberculosis*

Epidem: 80% of male genital TB is assoc with coexistent renal disease (Rev Infec Dis 1985;7:511). Epididymal disease usually develops in young sexually active males; up to 70% have a previous hx of TB (BJU 1989;64:305)

Pathophys: Epididymis appears to be blood-borne; usually starts in globus minor, which has greatest blood supply; may be assoc with renal disease, but not universal. Epididymal disease may be first and presenting symptom of GU TB. Testis: Almost always secondary to infection of the epididymis; 11% pts have renal lesion at autopsy (Urology 1982;20:43). May affect penis, epididymis, seminal vesicle, and prostate

Cmplc: Prostatic abscess (Aust NZ J Med 2000;30:94)

Sx: Painful testis/epididymis

Si: Draining scrotal sinus, scrotal swelling, tender testis/epididymis, nodular prostate, tender prostate, decreased volume of ejaculate

DiffDx: Epididymo-orchitis, prostate cancer, prostatitis

Lab: UA, c + s as for renal TB; culture of draining sinus for TB

Xray: KUB may show calcification of epididymis, prostate

Rx: Chemotherapy as for renal TB; epididymectomy if gross destruction/abscess formation of epididymis

5.4 GENITAL FILARIASIS

Cause: *Wuchereria bancrofti* accounts for 90% of cases. *Brugia malayi* and *B. timori* cause remainder. *Onchocerca volvulus*, a nonlymphatic parasite, can infect humans

Epidem: Transmitted by mosquitoes, take a long time to mature—up to a yr for onset of symptoms. 2-wk maturation in insect; infect via puncture holes; males and females in lymphatics produce microfilarial worms that migrate to peripheral blood in diurnal fashion, where ingested by insect and complete cycle. Found primarily in tropical areas. Large number of pts infected with filariae remain asx permanently (Lymphology 1976;9:11)

Pathophys: Adults block lymphatics, fibrotic nodules form about them in lymphatics or in subcutaneous locations (*Onchocerca*). Antigen-specific suppressor cells produced cause filaremia (Nejm 1982;307:144)

Sx: Onset may be delayed to 5+ yr after leave area. Local swelling and redness of skin where microfilaria enter; fever. Pts with filarial fever sustain episodic fevers, lymphangitis, lymphadenitis, funiculoepididymitis, transient edema, small acute hydroceles, and are typically amicrofilaremic. Pts with chronic pathology have chronic hydroceles, fixed edema, elephantiasis, chyluria, lymph scrotum

Crs: Chronic

Lab: Findings of *Brugia* or *Wuchereria* microfilaria in peripheral blood, chylous urine, or hydrocele fluid are diagnostic. 40% pos thin smears; thick smears better, or spin crit and look at buffy-coat smear under low power; eosinophilia. Specific serodiagnostic tests for *W. bancrofti* infection at CDC and ELISA for IgG4 ab against recombinant filarial ag appear promising (Am J Trop Med Hyg 1994;50:727)

Pathol: Bx of lymphatics/skin nodules (*Onchocerca*) shows adults

Serol: Positive

Rx: (Nejm 1985;313:133). Diethylcarbamazine (DEC). With high microfilarial counts start with low doses of DEC (3 mg/kg body weight/d), increase gradually to avoid severe sxs. Otherwise, 6 mg/kg body weight/d for total course of 72 mg/kg body weight for *W. bancrofti* and 4 mg/kg body weight/d for total of 60 mg/kg body weight for *B. malayi* (Campbell's Urology

1998;7(22):733–778; Acta Trop 1981;38:217). For genital
elephantiasis: Surgical rx to remove edematous and fibrotic tissue

5.5 FOURNIER'S GANGRENE (NECROTIZING FASCIITIS)

Semin Med 1984;4:69; 1983;3:345; Surg Gynecol Obstet 1990;170:49

Cause: Multiple organisms including aerobes (*E. coli*, *Klebsiella*,
enterococci) and anaerobes (*Bacteroides*, *Fusobacterium*,
Clostridium) (Surg Gynecol Obstet 1990;1970:49; AUA Update
Series 1986;5:6)

Epidem: Predisposing factors include DM, local trauma, paraphimosis,
periurethral extravasation of urine, perirectal or perianal
infections, and surgery such as circumcision or herniorrhaphy

Pathophys: Infection most commonly arises from the skin, urethra, or
rectal regions. Bacteria probably pass through Buck's fascia of the
penis and spread along the dartos fascia of the scrotum and penis,
Colles' fascia of the perineum, and Scarpa's fascia of the anterior
abdominal wall

Sx: Pain and malaise

Si: Fever, tachycardia, hypotension, crepitus, gangrene, swelling,
erythema of affected tissues

Crs: Onset usually abrupt and rapidly fulminating. Mortality rate of 20%
(Surg Gynecol Obstet 1990;170:49; BJU 1990;65:524). Higher
mortality in DM, alcoholics, and those with colorectal sources

Cmplc: May require urinary diversion and/or fecal diversion; may
require subsequent procedures to provide skin coverage of affected
areas

DiffDx: Perineal abscess

Lab: CBC, electrolytes, BUN and creatinine, type & cross

Xray: Plain film of abdomen may demonstrate subcutaneous air; scrotal
US may also demonstrate air

Rx: Fluid resuscitation, IV abx (combination of ampicillin plus
sulbactam or third-generation cephalosporin, such as ceftriaxone
plus gentamicin plus clindamycin). Once resuscitated, emergent
surgical debridement. Often need subsequent debridement in next
24 to 48 h. Extensive tissue coverage is often needed when the
infection is eradicated

5.6 CYSTADENOMA OF EPIDIDYMIS

Cause: Benign lesion originating from efferent ducts (Cancer 1976;37:1831)

Epidem: May be seen in Von Hippel–Lindau disease; bilateral lesions in 1/3 of cases, most often noted in young adults; may present with infertility

Pathophys: Benign epithelial hyperplasia

Sx: Minimal or no discomfort

Si: Enlarged epididymis

DiffDx: Testicular neoplasm, particularly teratoma

Xray: Scrotal US: Epididymal mass that is partially cystic

Rx: Epididymectomy

5.7 ADENOMATOID TUMOR

Cause: Benign neoplasm of adnexal structures. Possible etiologies: Reaction to injury/inflammation, mesothelial or endothelial origin (Campbell's Urology 1998;7(78):2411–2452)

Epidem: Most common of paratesticular tumors. Majority in head or tail of epididymis but occurs in testicular tunics and spermatic cord. Males in 20s–30s

Pathophys: Histopathology: Presence of vacuoles within epithelial cells

Si: Extratesticular solid mass, does not transilluminate

DiffDx: Malignant lesion, epididymal cyst

Xray: Scrotal US: Solid mass, typically in epididymis

Rx: Surgical excision

5.8 EPIDERMOID CYST

Cause: Benign neoplasm of the testis

Epidem: 1–2% of all testis tumors (Cancer 1981;47:577; BJU 1994;73:436). 50% occur in 20s; remainder between teens and 30s. Rarely bilateral (World J Urol 1984;2:76). Right side > left (1.27:1) (BJU 1994;73:436)

Pathophys: Tumor may represent a monolayer teratoma, but benign clinical behavior and not assoc with testicular intraepithelial neoplasia (Campbell's Urology 1998;7(78):2411–2452)

Sx: Usually painless

Si: Painless nodule/cyst

Crs: Benign lesion rarely coexists with malignant solid teratomatous elements. No case of local recurrence or mets (Urology 1993;41:75; BJU 1986;58:55)

DiffDx: Other testicular neoplasms

Lab: Serum markers: AFP, beta-HCG, and LDH if dx uncertain

Xray: Scrotal US: Well-circumscribed intratesticular cyst with hypoechoic center and circumferential echogenic whorls that do not shadow (Urology 1993;41:75)

Rx: Radical orchiectomy, but if confident of preoperative dx, then local incision. Bx adjacent testicular tissue to assess for testicular intraepithelial neoplasia to r/o mature teratoma (BJU 1993;71:612)

5.9 TESTIS CANCER—GERM CELL

Cause: May be congenital. Abnl of chromosome 12 identified in pts with testis cancer (Eur Urol 1993;23:23; Lancet 1982;2:1349). Alterations in tumor suppressor genes p53 and p16 have occurred (Proc Am Ass Cancer Res 1996;37:586; J Urol 1994;152:418)

Epidem: Most common malignancy in males aged 15–35 yr. Incidence is 6 per 100,000 men per yr and appears to be increasing (Int J Cancer 1996;65:723). 7–10% of pts with testicular cancer have history of UDT (Br J Hosp Med 1970;4:25). 2–3% of testicular tumors are bilateral

Pathophys: Testicular tumors may be divided into germ cell and nongerm cell tumors. Germ cell tumors account for 90–95% of all primary testicular tumors. Seminoma most common germ cell tumor in adults; yolk sac tumors most common in children. 40% of germ cells tumors are seminoma, 20–25% are embryonal carcinoma, 25–30% are teratocarcinoma, 5–10% are teratoma, and 1% are pure choriocarcinoma (Presti J. Testicular cancer: An overview. In: Crawford ED, Sakti D, eds. Current Genitourinary Cancer Surgery, 2nd ed. Baltimore: Williams & Wilkins, 1997:445–553). Pts may present with mixed germ cell tumors.

Nongerm cell tumors include Leydig cell tumors, Sertoli cell tumors, and gonadoblastomas. Secondary tumors of testis include lymphoma, leukemia, and metastatic (from prostate, lung, gastrointestinal tract, melanoma, kidney)

Staging Systems for Germ Cell Tumors

Skinner/Walter Reed		TNM	
A/I	Confined to testis	T1	Confined to testis
B/II	Retroperitoneum only	T2	Beyond tunica albuginea
B1/IIa	<6 positive nodes, all <2 cm	T3	Rete testis, epididymis
B2/IIb	>6 nodes, or any node >2 cm	T4a	Invasion of cord
B3/IIc	Bulky disease, >5 cm	T4b	Scrotal wall
C/III	Disease beyond retroperitoneum		
		N0	No nodes
		N1	One ipsilateral node <2 cm
		N2	Multiple nodes or one >2 cm
		N3	Nodes >5 cm

(Campbell's Urology 1998;7:2419–2420)

Sx: Pt may be asx or may present with pain or other sx of mets

Si: Palpable firm testis mass, reactive hydrocele, lower extremity edema with extensive adenopathy

Crs: If untreated, will met. Choriocarcinoma tends to met via a hematogenous route, the remainder via lymph nodes. Right-sided testicular tumors tend to met initially to interaorto-caval nodes, while left-sided tumors met to para-aortic retroperitoneal lymph nodes. Prior inguinal or scrotal surgery alters route of met spread

Cmplc: Cmplc assoc with RPLND incl ejaculatory failure, lymphocele, chylous ascites, intestinal adhesions, ureteral and vascular injury (AUA Update Series 1993;16:122). Cmplc assoc with chemotherapy incl bleomycin, pulmonary fibrosis, alopecia myelosuppression, renal insufficiency; cisplatin, renal insufficiency, N/V, neuropathy; etoposide (VP-16), myelosuppression, alopecia, renal insufficiency, leukemia

DiffDx: Intratesticular cyst, testis torsion, epididymitis, epidiymo-orchitis, hydrocele, hernia, hematoma, epidermoid or dermoid cyst

Lab: Beta-HCG elevated in pts with choriocarcinoma and may be elevated with embryonal carcinoma and seminoma. Beta-HCG produced by syncytiotrophoblast cells. Elevated beta-HCG may be seen with other malignancies including those of liver, pancreas, stomach, breast, kidney, and bladder, and may also be elevated in pts who smoke marijuana (Hematol Oncol Clin North Am 1991;5:1245). Serum half-life is 24–36 h. AFP may be produced by pure embryonal carcinoma, teratocarcinoma, yolk sac tumor, and mixed tumors but is not produced by pure choriocarcinoma or pure seminoma (Cancer 1980;45:1755,2166). This may be elevated in pts with lung, gastric, pancreatic, and hepatocellular cancers as well as liver disease (Hematol Oncol Clin North Am 1991;5:1245; GE 1983;65:530). Serum half-life is 5–7 d. LDH may be elevated with testicular tumors but its sens and specif are limited. Elevated levels may suggest extensive or bulky disease, and posttreatment increases indicate relapse (Semin Urol Oncol 1996;14:13; Urol Clin North Am 1993;20:67)

Xray: Scrotal US may help confirm presence of intratesticular mass. PA and lat chest xrays indicated in all pts except for those with abnl abdominal CT, in which case a chest CT is indicated (J Urol 1993;150:874). CT of abdomen/pelvis are part of staging workup in all pts to assess for lymphadenopathy. CT accuracy of 70–80% and a false neg rate of 23–44% (Urol Int 1988;443:198; Br J Radiol 1986;59:131; J Urol 1982;127:715)

Rx: Initial rx is serum labs, chest xray, and CT of abdomen/pelvis if they can be obtained promptly. Radical inguinal orchiectomy is performed. Subsequent rx based on clinical stage, tumor histology, and status of tumor markers (Oncology 1997;2:717). See Fig. 5–1 for treatment algorithms. Survival rate 95% and up (Urol Clin North Am 1998;25:397; Oncology 1997;11:717)

5.10 LEYDIG CELL TUMORS

Cause: Unknown. Appears to have no assoc with UDT

Epidem: 1–3% of testis tumors (Am J Surg Pathol 1985;9:177; Cancer 1975;35:1184; Cancer 1973;32:1186). Males age 20–60 yr, 25% occurring before puberty, 97% unilateral (Am J Surg Pathol 1985;9:177), 10% malignant, usually after 6th decade of life (Am J Surg Pathol 1985;9:177)

Pathophys: Histology: Reinke crystals. Criteria for malignancy are mets (Histopathol 1998;33:361)

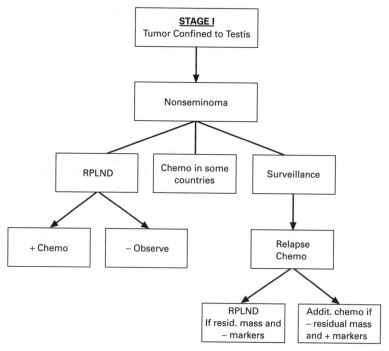

Figure 5–1. Treatment algorithm for nonseminomatous germ cell tumors of testis. A. Stage I.

Sx: 20% have pain (Am J Surg Pathol 1985;9:177). May have impotence, decreased libido, gynecomastia (Am J Surg Pathol 1985;9:177)

Si: In prepubertal boys: Isosexual precocity, prominent external genitalia, masculine voice, hair growth (Nejm 1999;341:1763), testicular enlargement. Most adults have no endocrine manifestations; 20–25% have feminizing effects (Cancer 1975;35:1184)

DiffDx: Other testicular neoplasms; in prepubertal cases r/o CAH; feminizing adrenocortical disorders, Klinefelter's syndrome, other feminizing testicular disorders

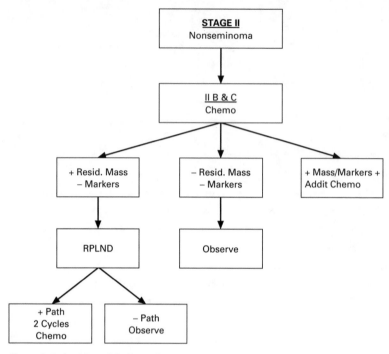

Figure 5–1. (*continued*) B. Stage II.

Lab: In prepubertal cases: Increased serum testosterone, ± elevated 17-ketosteroids. In adults may see increase in urinary and plasma estrogens, low gonadotropin and testosterone levels (Nejm 1999;341:1763)

Xray: Scrotal US: Intratesticular lesion, may be bilateral. MRI for detecting small nonpalpable lesions not identified on US (Clin Pediatr 1990;29:414)

Rx: Radical inguinal orchiectomy. If question of malignancy, CT of abdomen/pelvis for nodes. Virilizing and feminizing effects are to some extent irreversible

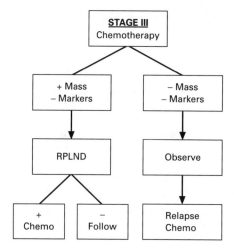

Figure 5–1. (*continued*) C. Stage III.

5.11 SERTOLI CELL TUMORS

Cause: Unknown. Majority occur in normal testes, but may occur in UDTs

Epidem: <1% of all testicular tumors, 10% malignant, 1/3 in pts ≥12 yr. Large cell calcifying assoc with Carney complex (myxoma, adrenocortical hyperplasia, pituitary tumor, skin pigmentation) and Peutz–Jeghers syndrome (Urology 1998;52:520; Am J Surg Pathol 1997;21:1271; Am J Clin Pathol 1980;74:607)

Pathophys: Histology: Epithelial elements resembling Sertoli cells, varying amounts of stroma, presence of mets is criteria for malignancy

Sx: May be painful or painless

Si: Testicular mass, ± gynecomastia

DiffDx: Leydig cell tumor

Lab: May note increased plasma testosterone in patients with virilization (Cancer 1975;35:1184)

Xray: Scrotal US: Intratesticular mass. If question of mets, CT of abdomen/pelvis, chest xray, bone scan

Rx: Radical orchiectomy. If malignant and enlarged nodes, RPLND
(Cancer 1968;22:8)

5.12 CARCINOID OF TESTIS

Cause: Malignant neoplasm
Epidem: Testis is infrequent site. May be site of metastasis also
Pathophys: To establish dx of primary, r/o lesion elsewhere (J Urol
1981;125:255). Histopathol: Identical to insular type of carcinoid
found in the intestine derived from the midgut (J Urol
1976;116:821). Primary carcinoid of testis may represent
unilateral development of a teratoma or may develop from
argentaffin cells within the testis (J Urol 1976;116:821)
Sx: Painless
Si: Slow-growing testicular enlargement
DiffDx: Other germ cell and nongerm cell tumors of the testis
Lab: Serum: AFP and beta-HCG are normal; 24-h urine for 5-HIAA
Xray: Scrotal US: Intratesticular lesion
Rx: Radical orchiectomy: If testicular primary, all that is necessary
(J Urol 1981;125:255; J Urol 1977;118:777)

5.13 GONADOBLASTOMA (TUMOR OF DYSGENETIC GONADS)

Cause: Occurs mostly in pts with gonadal dysgenesis
Epidem: 0.5% of all testis neoplasms. Affects all age groups, majority
males <30 yr
Pathophys: Histopathol: 3 elements: Sertoli cells, interstitial cells, germ
cells in varying proportions. Call–Exner bodies; Y chromosome in
almost all pts, 46 XY and 45X0/46 XY most common (Hum
Pathol 1991;22:884). 4/5 patients with gonadoblastoma are
phenotypic females, remainder phenotypic males (Cancer
1970;25:1340)
Si: In phenotypic females: Small breasts, hypoplastic internal genitalia,
± clitoral enlargement and streak gonads. In phenotypic male:

Gynecomastia, hypospadias, some internal female genitalia, dysgenetic testes

Crs: Invasive germinoma (seminoma); other germ cell tumors may also develop

DiffDx: Other testis neoplasms

Rx: Radical orchiectomy. Due to high incidence of bilateral disease (50%), contralateral gonadectomy indicated. If seminoma or other germ cell tumors identified, full staging evaluation indicated

5.14 LYMPHOMA OF THE TESTIS

Cause: May be manifestation of primary extranodal disease, initial manifestation of clinically occult nodal disease, or later manifestation of disseminated nodal lymphoma (Campbell's Urology 1998;7(78):2443)

Epidem: 2% of malignant tumors of testis in males <50 yr, 25% of those in older males (J Urol 1977;118:1004; BMJ 1963;2:891). Median age 60 yr. Bilateral in 50% pts, simultaneous in 10%, metachronously in remainder (Campbell's Urology 1998;7(78):2443). Primary lymphoma of testis may occur in children

Pathophys: Histology: Usually intermediate to high-grade B cell (J Urol 1996;155:943), diffuse replacement of the testis. Mets similar to germ cell tumors

Sx: 1/4 pts with generalized constitutional sx incl weight loss, weakness, anorexia

Si: Enlarged painless testis

Crs: Poor prognosis if generalized disease within 1 yr after dx. Pts with poorly differentiated lymphocytic types tend to survive longer than those with histiocytic. Pts with disease apparently confined to testis may live as long as 87 mo (Cancer 1981;48:2095). No evidence of systemic disease 1 yr after chemotherapy indicates high probability of cure

DiffDx: Other testicular neoplasms

Lab: CBC with peripheral smears, bone marrow studies

Xray: Scrotal US: Diffuse infiltration by the tumor (Radiation Med 1996;14:121). Chest xray, bone scan, CT, possibly liver/spleen scan

Rx: Radical orchiectomy and referral to oncologist

5.15 LEUKEMIA OF THE TESTIS

Cause: Testis is prime initial site of relapse in boys with ALL
Epidem: 8% incidence in children with ALL (Cancer 1975;35:1203)
Pathophys: Leukemic infiltration occurs in interstitial spaces, with
   destruction of tubules by infiltration in advanced cases (Campbell's
   Urology 1998;7(78):2411–2452)
Sx: Often painless
Si: Enlarged testis, may be bilateral, scrotal discoloration
Crs: Interval from testis involvement to death ranges from 5 to 27 mo,
   median 9 mo (Campbell's Urology 1998;7(78):2411–2444)
DiffDx: Other testicular neoplasms
Xray: Diffuse testicular enlargement
Rx: Bx of testis for dx. Testis XRT: 2000cGy with reinstitution of
   adjunctive chemotherapy or reinduction therapy for children who
   relapse in testis while on chemotherapy

5.16 SECONDARY TUMORS OF THE TESTIS: LYMPHOMA, LEUKEMIA, METASTATIC

Cause: Neoplasia
Epidem:
   Lymphoma: Accounts for 5% of all testis tumors, most common
      secondary neoplasm of testis, most frequent of all testis tumors in
      males >50 yr. Median age 60 yr
   Leukemia: 8% incidence of extramedullary involvement of testis in
      children with ALL (Cancer 1975;35:1203)
   Metastatic: Usually occurs in 50s and 60s
Pathophys:
   Lymphoma: See 5.14
   Leukemia: See 5.15
   Metastatic: Most common primary sources include prostate, lung, GI
      tract, melanoma, renal
Sx:
   Lymphoma: Generalized constitutional sx of weight loss, weakness,
      and anorexia

Leukemia: Often asx

Metastatic: Sx related to primary disease and other sites of mets

Si:

Lymphoma: Diffuse testicular enlargement; 50% pts have bilateral tumors, simultaneously in 10% and metachronously in the rest, adenopathy may be present

Leukemia: Diffuse testicular enlargement, bilateral in 50% cases; may have scrotal discoloration

Metastatic: Solid testicular mass; may be multiple

Crs:

Lymphoma: See 5.14

Leukemia: See 5.15

Cmplc: R/o orchitis or primary testis tumor; surgery and/or chemotherapy may impair fertility

Lab: Serum AFP, beta-HCG, and LDH. Lymphoma: CBC, peripheral smears, bone marrow bx. Leukemia: CBC, bone marrow bx. Metastatic: As dictated by primary lesion

Xray:

Lymphoma: Chest xray, bone scan, CT

Metastatic: CT to evaluate for additional mets

Rx:

Lymphoma: See 5.14

Leukemia: See 5.15

Metastatic: Testis bx if suspect, rx as per primary cancer

5.17 LEIOMYOSARCOMA OF THE SPERMATIC CORD

Cause: Malignant neoplasm

Epidem: Rare. 10% of spermatic cord sarcomas in adults (Urology 1984;23:187)

Pathophys: Originates from smooth muscle of spermatic cord vessels. 3 patterns of spread: high risk of local recurrence and extension, hematogenous spread to lung, and lymph mets such as para-aortic lymph nodes (J Urol 1991;146:342; Urology 1984;23:187; J Urol 1981;126:611)

Sx: Painless

Si: Firm, intrascrotal mass that does not involve testis or epididymis, gradually enlarging

DiffDx: Other benign and malignant neoplasms of the cord

Lab: AFP and beta-HCG to r/o testis neoplasm

Xray: Scrotal US: Paratesticular solid mass. MRI: Specif 88% for intrascrotal lesions (Fortschr Roentgenstr 1991;155:436). CT abdomen/pelvis to r/o retroperitoneal adenopathy. Chest xray to r/o lung mets

Rx: Radical (inguinal) orchiectomy (Urology 1984;23:187; J Urol 1981;126:611; Br J Urol 1981;53:193). RPLND indicated for enlarged nodes on CT scan. Adjuvant chemotherapy and XRT advantageous in high-grade sarcomas (J Urol 1991;146:342; Urology 1986;27:28; Urology 1984;23:187). Adjuvant XRT helps reduce local recurrence (Int J Urol 1999;6:536). Poor prognosis with recurrent disease

5.18 TESTIS RUPTURE

Eur Urol 1994;25:119; J Urol 1993;150:1143)

Cause: Blunt or penetrating trauma

Epidem: May be accidental or self-induced

Pathophys: Tear of the tunica albuginea allows for extrusion of seminiferous tubules

Si: Scrotal ecchymosis/hematoma, inability to fully palpate the testis

Sx: Pain

X-ray: Scrotal US: Overall accuracy for detection of traumatic testis rupture; specif, 75%; sens, 64%; pos predictive value, 77.8%, neg predictive value, 60% (J Urol 1993;150:1834)

Rx: Immediate exploration if rupture suspected. Debride necrotic and extruded tissue, close tunica albuginea, drain, and 7 d abx

5.19 VARICOCELE

Cause: Dilatation of the pampiniform plexus of veins around testis may be secondary to anatomic considerations (left testicular vein entering into left renal vein), incompetent venous valves, or "nutcracker phenomenon" (compression of the left renal vein between the superior mesenteric artery and aorta) (J Urol 1980;124:833) or obstruction of the inferior vena cava

Epidem: Rare prior to puberty. Left side (90%) > right; may be bilateral. About 16% adolescents have a varicocele (Pediatr Med Chir 1993;15:159). Approximately 40% men seen for infertility will have a varicocele and >50% have improvement in semen analysis after varicocelectomy (J Androl 1986;7:147)

Pathophys: Deleterious effects on testis may be secondary to elevated intrascrotal temperature as a result of pooling of warm venous blood (Fertil Steril 1988;49:199; J Urol 1988;139:207). Other possible theories incl reflux of adrenal and renal metabolites from renal vein (Fertil Steril 1974;25:88), decreased blood flow (J Clin Invest 1981;68:39), and hypoxia (J Androl 1985;6:117). Changes may affect both testes (J Clin Invest 1981;68:39)

Cmplc: Infertility

Si: "Bag of worms" in ipsilateral scrotum, decreased ipsilateral testicular size

Sx: Scrotal discomfort

Lab: Semen analysis: Decreased motility most common, 65% with decreased sperm concentration (<20 million/cc), "stress pattern"— increased numbers of amorphous cells and immature germ cells (Fertil Steril 1965;16:735). Nl testosterone, occasionally increased FSH (Fertil Steril 1975;26:1006)

Xray: Scrotal US: Most accurate way to assess testicular size. Renal US for acute right varicocele: R/o obstruction of inferior vena cava

Rx: Adolescent: Rx indicated for clinically detectable varicocele assoc with ipsilateral decreased testicular size (J Urol 1988;139:562; 1987;137:475). Adult: Rx if male is infertile with abnl semen analysis. Improvement in seminal parameters noted in 70% after repair; motility is most common factor improved followed by density and morphology (J Urol 1986;136:609; 1979;121:435). Repair of large varicocele assoc with significantly greater improvement in semen quality than small varicocele (J Urol

1996;155:1287). Goal of rx is ligation or occlusion of the dilated veins; may be accomplished via inguinal or subinguinal approach, retroperitoneal or laparoscopic approach, or via radiologic occlusion technique. Risks of surgery: recurrence, hydrocele, injury to testicular artery. Conception rates after repair average 40–50% (J Urol 1986;136:609; 1979;121:435; Urology 1977;10:446)

5.20 MALE INFERTILITY

Cause: Structural, chromosomal, infectious (genital tract and postpubertal mumps orchitis), medication/drug-induced, immunologic, chemotherapy and XRT-induced, and obstructive causes. Infertility may be due to incorrect coital habits, abnl sperm count (oligospermia, azoospermia), abnl sperm motility (asthenospermia), abnl sperm morphology, and ejaculatory dysfunction

Epidem: Approximately 20% cases of infertility due entirely to a male factor. Additional 30% involve both male and female factors (Fertil Steril 1991;56:192)

Eval: History and physical examination: Evaluate coital habits, use of lubricants that may affect sperm motility (Lubafax, K-Y Jelly, Keri Lotion, Surgilube, and saliva) (Fertil Steril 1987;47:882; 1982;38:721; 1975;26:872; Am J Obstet Gynecol 1972;113:88), recent febrile illness (may impair fertility for 1–3 mo), medications, surgical hx, trauma. Assess secondary sex characteristics, testis size and position, presence of vas, palpate epididymis, r/o hypospadias, assess for varicocele, DRE to r/o seminal vesicle enlargement

Lab: Semen analysis: 2 d of abstinence and brought to lab within 2 h of collection. Nl semen parameters: Volume 1.5–5.0 mL, total sperm count >50 million (≥20 million/cc), motility >50%, forward progression >2, morphology >50% nl sperm morphology by standard criteria or >14% nl forms by strict criteria (Campbell's Urology 1998;7(4):1287–1330). If history and physical supportive or sperm density <5–10 million sperm/mL, then check LH, FSH, and testosterone

   Absent or Low-Volume Ejaculate: Check postintercourse urine for sperm. If no ejaculate and urine shows >5–10 sperm/hpf, suggests retrograde ejaculation. If low-volume ejaculate and urine shows more sperm than in ejaculate, also suggests retrograde ejaculation. May rx retrograde ejaculation with ephedrine sulfate (25–50 mg qid), pseudoephedrine HCl (60 mg qid), or imipramine HCl (25 mg bid). If no effect within 2 wk, success unlikely. If absent or low-volume ejaculate and no sperm present in urine, need TRUS of seminal vesicles and ejaculatory ducts to r/o congenital anomaly or obstruction. Ejaculatory duct obstruction may be treated with TUR. If TRUS is nl, testis bx to assess for spermatogenesis. If sperm present, further evaluation for physical or functional obstruction. If testis bx shows no sperm, check LH, FSH, and testosterone. If FSH is >2–3 × nl, with nl LH and testosterone and testes small suggests germ cell failure. Rx with artificial insemination or adoption. If FSH elevated, LH elevated, and testosterone nl or low, suggests testicular failure. If both FSH and LH low, further endocrine evaluation indicated for hypogonadotropic hypogonadism

Oligospermia: Rarely seen as an isolated finding on semen analysis. In severe cases of oligospermia, check LH, FSH, and testosterone; if these are abnl, need full endocrine evaluation. If lab nl, pt is a candidate for assisted reproduction or empiric medical rx (clomiphene citrate)

Asthenospermia: May be secondary to prolonged abstinence periods, genital tract infection, antisperm abs, partial ductal obstruction, or idiopathic causes. Check antisperm ab assay; if pos may proceed with immunosuppression or assisted reproduction. If antisperm ab assay neg, r/o pyospermia; if no pyospermia, r/o obstruction, varicocele, heat, systemic illness, and consider viability assay. Antisperm abs present in 60% after vasectomy (Fertil Steril 1971;22:629). Testicular torsion and trauma may lead to development of antisperm abs

A variety of syndromes (Kallman's, fertile eunuch, isolated FSH deficiency, Prader–Willi) are assoc with deficiencies of gnRH, LH, and FSH. Rx consists of restoring the deficiencies. Genetic anomalies assoc with infertility include Klinefelter's syndrome (XXY male), XX male, androgen abnormalities (deficiency in androgen synthesis, conversion of testosterone to DHT, androgen receptor abnormalities), and Noonan's syndrome (46 XY)

UDT assoc with decreased sperm concentrations. 50% of pts with bilateral UDTs and 25–30% of pts with unilateral UDT will have sperm concentrations <12–20 million/mL (J Urol 1989;142:749;

Nejm 1976;295:15). The higher the UDT, the more severe the testicular dysfunction

Varicocele is the most common surgically treatable cause of infertility

Anejaculation may occur in pts with retroperitoneal surgery, spinal cord injury, MS, transverse myelitis, and DM. Rx with vibratory stimulation or electroejaculation (J Urol 1990;344a). Congenital hypoplasia or absence of the vas deferens is manifested as low-volume azoospermia with a testis bx demonstrating spermatogenesis. Rx with epididymal sperm aspiration and intracytoplasmic sperm injection (ICSI)

Assisted Reprod:

Intrauterine Insemination (IUI): Pregnancy 7–19% per stimulated cycle and 0.2–22% in nonstimulated cycles (Hum Reprod 1994;9:2022; Fertil Steril 1992;58:995; 1987;47:441; 1986;6:673; Obstet Gynecol 1983;82:780)

In Vitro Fertilization: Fertilization rates lower with male factor infertility. Live birth rates average 16.6% per egg retrieval cycle for male factor couples compared to 21.5% for nonmale-factor couples (Feril Steril 1995;64:13). Intracytoplasmic sperm injection (ICSI): Pregnancy rates of 25–35% per egg retrieval cycle have been reported (Hum Reprod 1994;9:2051; 1993;8:1061)

6 Diseases of the Prostate

6.1 PROSTATITIS

Cause: Bacterial and nonbacterial etiologies

Epidem: Prostatitis affects up to 50% of men at some point in their lives. Affects men of all ages. (Current Opin Urol 1998;8:33). About 8% of all urology visits in U.S. related to prostatitis (National Ambulatory Medical Care Survey 1992). Only about 6–8% of men with "prostatitis" will have bacterial prostatitis (Urology 1990;36(5 suppl):13)

Pathophys:

NIH classification and definitions of prostatitis:

I.   Acute bacterial prostatitis

II. Chronic bacterial prostatitis: recurrent infection

III. Chronic abacterial prostatitis/chronic pelvic pain syndrome: No demonstrable infection

IIIA. Inflammatory chronic pelvic pain syndrome: wbc present in semen/expressed prostatic secretions or voided bladder urine (VB3)

IIIB. Noninflammatory chronic pelvic pain syndrome: no wbc noted in semen/expressed prostatic secretions or VB3

IV. Asymptomatic inflammatory prostatitis: Detected by prostate bx or presence of wbcs in prostatic secretions during evaluation for other disorders (Jama 1999;282:236)

Organisms isolated in acute and chronic bacterial prostatitis are same as those causing UTI (Techniques Urol 1995;1:162). *E. coli* accounts for 80% of prostatic infections; other gram-negative organisms (*Pseudomonas aeruginosa, Serratia, Klebsiella proteus*) account for 10–15% of infections. Enterococci identified in

5–10% cases of prostatitis (Urology 1997;49:809). Role of *Chlamydia trachomatis* in prostatitis is controversial. Etiology of acute bacterial prostatitis is often due to reflux of infected urine into prostatic ducts that drain into posterior urethra (BJU 1974;46:537; BJU 1982;54:729). Inflammation and edema may lead to occlusion of these ducts, trapping bacteria within, leading to chronic bacterial prostatitis (Urology 1997;49:809). Intraprostatic urinary reflux, causing a "chemical" prostatitis, may play a role in etiology of nonbacterial prostatitis (Urology 1987;30:183)

Sx: Urinary frequency and urgency, dysuria, malaise, pain in perineum, groin, testes, back, suprapubic area

Si: Fever/chills if acute bacterial, decreased urine flow rate, nocturia; tender, boggy, or firm prostate on DRE

DiffDx: Distal ureteral calculus, Müllerian remnant, urethral stricture, BPH, seminal vesicle cyst, prostatic cyst, IC, bladder cancer, urachal remnant, hernia, ejaculatory duct cyst, depression/stress, spinal stenosis, mesenteric cyst, fibromyalgia

Lab: Meares–Stamey test is gold standard for dx of bacterial prostatitis. After cleansing and retraction of foreskin, pt voids first 10 mL into sterile container (VB1), then collects midstream 5–10 mL (VB2), then prostatic massage performed collect expressed prostatic secretions and review under microscope and collect first 10 mL of urine after massage (VB3). Modification of Nickels allows for simple testing with 91% sens and specif compared to Meares–Stamey technique. Modified technique: Collect midstream urine and perform prostatic massage, then collect postmassage urine and perform UA, c + s on both. Future studies include immunologic techniques to allow for ab screening of the expressed prostatic secretions or VB3 specimen for common prostatic pathogens and molecular biologic techniques using PCR to id bacterial gene products (Urology 1998;51:362)

Xray: Bladder scanner PVR to ensure complete bladder emptying. Uroflow helpful in pts with voiding complaints. Cystoscopy not indicated in most pts. Videourodynamics in pts with nonbacterial chronic prostatitis may demonstrate "spastic dysfunction" of bladder neck and prostatic urethra

Rx: Rx acute bacterial prostatitis with abx; typically fluoroquinolones for 6–12 wk. Tm/S may be used. Chronic bacterial prostatitis rx with abx for extended periods; in pts with frequent recurrent

infections long-term prophylactic abx may be employed.
Pts with chronic nonbacterial prostatitis may be treated as follows.
Category IIIA: Trial of broad-spectrum abx, alpha-blocker
therapy, anti-inflammatory agents,? finasteride if enlarged prostate,
prostatic massage (2–3 ×/wk), supportive therapy (counseling),
transurethral microwave therapy or phytotherapy. Category IIIB:
Alpha-blocker therapy, muscle relaxant, analgesics, biofeedback,
relaxation exercises, supportive therapy (counseling). Other
therapies: Sitz baths; avoidance of spices, caffeine, and alcohol.
Biofeedback has encouraging results in pts with noninflammatory
chronic pelvic pain syndrome (Curr Opin Urol 1996;6:53)

6.2 PROSTATIC ABSCESS

Cause: Bacterial infection

Epidem: Most cases occur in men in their 50s–60s but also has been
reported in infants (Rev Infect Dis 1988;10:239). Since the 1940s
the incidence has decreased and the causative organism has
changed. Prior to the 1940s, *Neisseria gonorrhoeae* accounted for
40% of cases; currently *E. coli* accounts for 70% of cases (Rev
Infect Dis 1988;10:239; Am J Surg 1931;11:334). Rarely, may
occur secondary to *Staphylococcus aureus* infection (J Urol
1986;136:1281). Increased risk in males with DM, chronic renal
failure on dialysis, immunocompromised and recent urethral
instrumentation, or requiring chronic indwelling catheters
(Rev Infect Dis 1988;10:239; J Urol 1986;136:1281)

Pathophys: Secondary to ascending urethral infection and intraprostatic
reflux of infected urine, which leads to acute bacterial prostatitis,
which in predisposed individuals may develop into a prostatic
abscess

Sx: Dysuria, frequency, perineal pain, low back pain

Si: Urinary retention, fever/chills, hematuria, urethral discharge. Prostate
may be fluctuant (16%), tender to palpation (35%), or enlarged
(75%) on DRE (Rev Infect Dis 1988;10:239)

Cx: Mortality rate of about 5% (Rev Infect Dis 1988;10:239)

DiffDx: Prostatitis, seminal vesiculitis

Lab: UA, c + s, CBC

Xray: CT scan or transrectal US helps to dx and serves as a guide for percutaneous aspiration for culture, drainage, and to evaluate response to rx

Rx: Abx specific for the organism and drainage. Drainage may be achieved percutaneously or via transurethral incision/resection

6.3 BENIGN PROSTATIC HYPERPLASIA (BPH)

Cause: Benign neoplasm of the prostate. Development requires a combination of testicular androgens and aging (J Androl 1991;12:356)

Epidem: Most common neoplastic condition affecting males. 30% prevalence by physical exam; at age 40–50, 35% of all men eventually will have sx requiring meds or surgery (Prostate 1996;6(suppl):67), and 50% over age 70

Pathophys: Hyperplastic tissue located centrally in periurethral portion of the prostate. All glandular and stromal elements of the normal prostate are involved to a variable degree in BPH. Sx do not necessarily correlate with the prostatic size (J Urol 1984;132:474; BJU 1981;53:613)

Sx: Urinary frequency, urinary urgency, feeling of incomplete emptying, nocturia, hesitancy, intermittent stream. AUA scoring system (Nejm 1995;332:99): 5 points = always, $4 = >^1/_2$ the time, $3 = {}^1/_2$ the time, $2 = <^1/_2$ the time, $= <^1/_5$ the time, 0 = never, for each of the following sx:

1. Incomplete emptying
2. Frequency >q2 h
3. Stop/start voiding
4. Urgency
5. Decreased flow
6. Strains to void
7. Nocturia, 0–5+ /noc

Classification: Mild = 0–7 total points, moderate = 8–18, severe = 19–35. Scoring system is helpful in assessing the severity of sx but is not specific for BPH

Si: Enlarged prostate, distended bladder, hematuria, incontinence, UTI, urinary retention. Prostate size: No standardized nomenclature for describing prostate size; commonly used: Normal gland is size of horse chestnut, 20 gm

1+ enlarged: About size of a plum; 25 gm, occupies $<1/4$ rectal lumen

2+ enlarged: About size of a lemon; 50 gm, fills $1/2$ of rectal lumen

3+ enlarged: About size of an orange; 75 gm, fills $3/4$ of rectal lumen

4+ enlarged: About size of a small grapefruit; ≥100 gm, fills fair amount of rectal lumen, difficult to completely feel prostate.

DRE tends to underestimate prostate size up to 40 gm (J Urol 1986;135:190)

Crs: 39% chance that men >60 yr will require surgery for BPH in next 20 yr (Urology 1991;38(suppl 1):4)

Cmplc: Urinary retention, renal insufficiency, chronic/recurrent UTI, gross hematuria, bladder stones, bladder calculi: no increased risk of prostate cancer except that incurred by age (Ann IM 1997;126:480)

DiffDx: (1) Other causes of BOO: Bladder neck obstruction, prostate cancer, Müllerian duct cysts, urethral stricture, urethral valves; (2) impaired detrusor contractility; (3) DH/DI; (4) inflammatory and infectious conditions including cystitis, carcinoma in situ of the bladder; (5) prostatitis syndromes including acute bacterial prostatitis, chronic prostatitis, nonbacterial prostatitis, prostatodynia, pelvic floor dysfunction

Lab: UA, c + s to r/o hematuria and infection; serum BUN and creatinine to evaluate renal function. Noninvasive: Peak urine flow rate (voided volume must be at least 150 cc to be reliable): >20 cc/sec nl, 15–20 cc/sec = mild, 10–15 cc/sec = moderate, <10 cc/sec+ = severe, not specific for BPH (Nejm 1995;332:99). Invasive: Urodynamic evaluation including flow rate, assessment of PVR, and CMG may be helpful in some patients; allows assessment of detrusor function

Xray: Renal/bladder US may be helpful to assess upper tracts and bladder emptying; IVP also may help assess upper tracts

Rx: (Nejm 1995;332:99). Rx primarily for quality of life. Criteria for intervention: Urinary retention, bilateral hydronephrosis with altered renal function, recurrent or chronic UTI, recurrent gross hematuria of prostatic origin, bladder calculi, pt desire

Medical: Avoid caffeine and alcohol. Alpha-blockers: Tone of bladder neck and prostate is thought to be autonomically controlled via alpha₁-adrenoreceptors (J Urol 1989;141:1283; J Urol 1983;130:275). Terazosin (Hytrin) (Nejm 1996;335:533): Start with 1 mg and increase sequentially to max of 5–10 mg po qd, improves flow within 2 wks (Med Let 1994;36:15). Doxazosin (Cardura): Start with 2 mg po qd, and increase to max of 8 mg po qd as tolerated. Both doxazosin and terazosin may cause postural hypotension and BP should be checked with each incremental dose. Tamsulosin (Flomax) (Med Let 1997;39:96): Daily dose of 0.4 or 0.8 mg ¹/₂ h after same meal each day, no titration necessary. All alpha-blockers have potential side effects of dizziness, nasal stuffiness, and ejaculatory dysfunction. 5-alpha-reductase inhibitor decreases plasma and intraprostatic dihydrotestosterone levels (Arch Androl 1982;9:56). Finasteride (Proscar) 5 mg po qd (Nejm 1998;338:612; Nejm 1994;330:120; Nejm 1992; 327:1185). Works best on large prostate glands. May take 6 mo–1 yr for maximal improvement in sx. If effective, may remain so for at least 5 yrs. Lowers PSA by 50% (Prostate 1993;22:31). Long-term finasteride use does not appear to affect histologic features of BPH (Urology 1999;32:696). With long-term (5 yr) rx, prevalence of ejaculatory disorder, impotence, and decreased libido was 2.7%, 9.6%, and 3.7%, respectively

Herbal Therapies: About 30 phytotherapeutic compounds used for BPH (Urology 1996;48:12): Saw palmetto plant extract, serenoa repens are most commonly used. Saw palmetto appears to improve urologic sxs and flow measures when compared to placebo and similar to that provided by finasteride (Jama;1998:280:1604). Long-term effects and effect on PSA need to be further evaluated

Surgical: TURP, still considered gold-standard, required in 10%, if retention and/or severe sx; cmplc = 4% incontinence, 5% impotence at 1 yr (Jama 1988;259:3010) but later VA study found incontinence and sexual dysfunction same in watchful waiting pts as in operated pts (Nejm 1995;332:75). Other risks: Bleeding requiring transfusion, retrograde ejaculation, urethral/bladder neck stricture. Suprapubic/retropubic prostatectomy useful in large prostate glands or when there is coexistent large bladder calculi. Transurethral microwave thermotherapy (Lancet 1993;341:14; BMJ 1993;306:1293) less effective than TURP, probably similar to medical therapy (Med Let 1996;38:53). Other options: Laser prostatectomy, incision best in small glands and those who wish to maintain antegrade ejaculation; prostatic urethral stenting;

transurethral needle ablation (TUNA), and transurethral
vaporization of the prostate

6.4 PROSTATE CANCER

Cause: Neoplasia. Estimated that 9% of all prostate cancers and
more than 40% of cases of early-onset disease are attributed
to autosomal dominant gene (Proc Natl Acad Sci USA
1993;89:3371). Abnormalities of chromosome 1 and the X
chromosome assoc with increased risk of prostate cancer (Am
J Hum Genet 1999;64:776; Nat Genet 1998;20:175; Am
J Hum Genet 1998;62:1416; Science 1996;274:1371). Plasma
concentrations of insulin-like growth factor-1 (IGF-1) assoc
with increased risk of developing prostate cancer (Science
1998;279:563). Decreased p27 (a cell-cycle inhibitor) reactivity
is assoc with higher Gleason grade, positive surgical margins,
seminal vesical involvement, and lymph node mets (Mod Pathol
1998;11:324)

Epidem: Most common form of noncutaneous cancer in males in the
U.S.; second leading cause of male cancer mortality. Prostate
cancer accounted for 30,000 deaths in 1999 (Oncology
2000;14:267). 95% of prostate cancer is diagnosed in men ages
45–89 yr (median, 72 yr) (Cancer J Clin 1995;45:8). Black males
living in the U.S. have a higher incidence rate than white males,
are routinely diagnosed with later-stage disease, and have lower
survival rates as compared to white men (J Natl Cancer Inst
1991;83:551). In the setting of familial disease, the risk of a man
developing prostate cancer depends on age of onset of prostate
cancer and number of affected relatives (J Urol 1993;150:797).
Other possible risk factors incl dietary fat (Cancer Res
1983;43(s):2397), cadmium exposure (Epidemiology 1990;1:107),
and vitamin D deficiency (Endocrinology 1995;136:20)

Pathophys: Tends to be found in peripheral portion of the prostate
gland. Multifocal in 85% of cases (Cancer 1972;30:5). 1/3 of
prostate cancers identified through early detection efforts with PSA
and DRE treated surgically have evidence of extracapsular spread,
poor differentiation on histology, large tumor volume, or distant
mets. Gleason grade is based on glandular pattern of tumor as

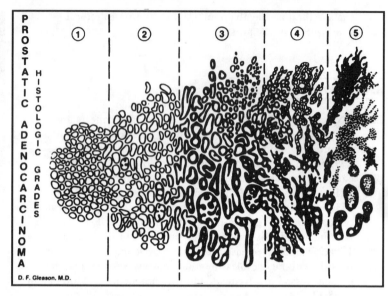

Figure 6–1. Gleason grade prostate cancer. (Reproduced with permission from Epstein JI. Pathology of adenocarcinoma of the prostate. In Walsh et al., eds. Campbell's urology, 7th ed. Philadelphia: Saunders, 1998:2499.)

identified under relatively low magnification and ranges from 1–5 (Fig. 6–1). Gleason sum (score) is the addition of the primary and secondary patterns present on microscopic examination and ranges from 2–10. Gleason scores ≥7 considered biologically aggressive tumors; those ≤4 are considered to have low aggressive potential. Tumor grade is strongest prognostic factor (Jama 1998;280:975). Tumor volume >0.5 cc is thought to be clinically significant (Oncology 2000;14:267)

Sx: Pts may present with obstructive voiding symptoms or bone pain from bony mets

Si: DRE may reveal a firm, hard, nontender mass (nodule)

Crs: Clinical course varies with age at dx, tumor grade, tumor stage, and volume of disease on presentation. Also affected by p27 reactivity. TNM staging of prostate cancer (N and M refer to the presence, absence, and extent of nodal and metastatic disease, respectively (BJU 1975;47:1):

T1 Clinically unapparent tumor, not palpable or visible by imaging
T1a Tumor found incidentally at TUR; <5% of tissue is cancerous
T1b Tumor found incidentally at TUR, >5% of tissue is cancerous
T1c Tumor identified by prostate needle bx because of elevated PSA
T2 Palpable tumor confined within the prostate
T2a Tumor involves half of a lobe or less
T2b Tumor involves > half of one lobe, but not both lobes
T2c Tumor involves both lobes
T3 Palpable tumor through prostate capsule and/or involving seminal vesicles
T3a Unilateral extracapsular extension
T3b Bilateral extracapsular extension
T3c Tumor invades seminal vesicle(s)
T4 Tumor is fixed or invades adjacent structures other than seminal vesicles
T4a Tumor invades bladder neck and/or external sphincter and/or rectum
T4b Tumor invades levator muscles and/or is fixed to pelvic wall

Cmplc: Local invasion, bone mets (often osteoblastic, but may be osteolytic), and other mets

Lab:

Chem: Acid phosphatase, prostatic fraction increased in 67% with metastatic disease; false pos with hepatic impairment (Nejm 1980;303:497).

PSA: A glycoprotein produced principally by the epithelial cells lining the prostatic acini and ducts. May be elevated in males with BPH and prostatitis. Age-adjusted PSA:

Age (y)	White	Black
40–49	0–2.5	0–2.0
50–59	0–3.5	0–4.0
60–69	0–3.5	0–4.5
70–79	0–3.5	0–5.5

(Nejm 1996;335(5):304–210). In range of 4–10.0, PSA lacks specif; about 75% of males with PSA in this range will not have prostate cancer (Jama 1998;279:1542). PSA velocity is the change in PSA/change in time. Some suggest that a rise of >0.75 ng/mL in a year is cause for concern (Jama 1992;267:2215). PSA density is the PSA/prostate volume. PSA density >0.15 is proposed as the threshold for performing a bx in males with PSA 4–10 and neg

DRE and neg TRUS, but this is not uniformly accepted (Urology 1994;43:44; J Urol 1994;152:2031; Urol Clin North Am 1993;20:653). Free/total PSA: The PSA exists in blood in two states, a free state and bound to plasma proteins. Pts with prostate cancer tend to have lower free/total PSA ratios. Ratios of 14–28% have been proposed as cut-offs (J Urol 1999;162:293)

Lab: Needle bx and histologic/cytologic grading

Xray: Transrectal US cannot exclude presence of prostate cancer, but is helpful in guiding prostate bxs. Bone scan, CT scan, and MRI are used in staging and follow-up of patients with prostate cancer, but are not indicated in all pts. In newly diagnosed prostate cancer, CT or MRI generally not necessary if PSA <25.0 ng/mL. Bone scan not necessary with clinically localized prostate cancer when PSA <10.0 ng/mL (Oncology 2000;14:267)

Other: BPLND may be omitted if PSA <10.0 ng/mL or if PSA <20.0 ng/mL and Gleason score ≤6 (Oncology 2000;14:267)

Rx:

Screening: Recommended by AUA that early detection of prostate cancer should be offered to asx males ≥50 yr who have estimated life expectancy of 10 yrs. Reasonable to offer testing at earlier age to males with defined risk factors, including first-degree relatives with prostate cancer and African-American males (Oncology 2000:14:267). In men with no cancer suspected on DRE and baseline PSA <2.0 ng/mL, PSA testing interval can be every 2 yr. If baseline PSA >2 ng/mL, PSA should be checked yrly (Jama 1997;277:1456)

Stage T1a: No rx if low Gleason score. If Gleason score ≥7 RRPX or XRT

Stage T1b, c, T2a, T2b, T2c: RRPX or XRT ± BPLND, depending upon PSA and Gleason score

Stage T3a,b, c: RRPX vs. XRT. Likelihood of pos lymph nodes higher

Stage T4a, b: XRT for local control; hormonal therapy

Metastatic Disease: Hormonal therapy, which is palliative. A VA study comparing early versus late hormonal therapy showed no survival advantage with early rx (Cancer 1973;32:1126)

Surgical Castration: Gold standard of endocrinologic rx of prostate cancer. Side effects incl loss of libido and potency, hot flashes, osteoporosis, fatigue, loss of muscle mass, anemia, weight gain

LHRH Agonists: After initial phase of stimulation (2–3 wk) lead to a suppression of LH and of testosterone production to castrate levels (Biochem Biophys Res Commun 1977;76:855). Commonly used agents include leuprolide (Med Let 1985;27:71; Nejm 1984;311:1281), buserelin (Nejm 1989;321:413), and goserelin (Med Let 1990;32:102). In pts with mets, a pure or steroidal antiandrogen should be instituted 1 wk prior to LHRH therapy to prevent biochemical and clinical flare. Side effects are the same as for surgical castration

Antiandrogens: Interfere with androgen action by binding to androgen receptor. Steroidal antiandrogens (CPA, megestrol acetate) suppress gonadotropins and lower plasma testosterone levels. Pure antiandrogens incl flutamide (Eulexin), nilutamide, and biclutamide (Casodex). Pure antiandrogens do not affect libido and potency. Nilutamide and biclutamide not indicated for monotherapy. Most commonly used in combination with the LHRH agonists for maximal androgen blockade. Side effects of pure antiandrogens include gynecomastia, abnormal liver function tests, diarrhea, and GI complaints (Urology 1988;31;312)

Bone Mets: Frequently used regimen is 300cGy of XRT in 10 divided doses. In pts with significant bony mets and pain, strontium 89 (metastron) or samarium 153 (Quadramet) may be helpful (Med Let 1997;39:83). Toxicity of these agents primarily hematologic

6.5 PROSTATIC CALCULI

Cause: Deposition of calcareous material on corpora amylacea; develop in the tissues or acini of the gland. May occur secondary to infections and may be assoc with ochronosis (Urology 1991;37:240)

Epidem: Rare in boys. Frequently identified in males over age 50. Often noted incidentally on routine x-rays. Composed of calcium phosphate trihydrate and carbonate (BJU 1974;46:533)

Sx: Usually asx. Sx may be secondary to BPH, urethral stricture, or prostatitis

Si: Calcification on plain film of abdomen and pelvis, may have terminal hematuria

Crs: Often asx

Cmplc: If infected, may lead to recurrent infection

DiffDx: Bladder calculi

Lab: UA, c + s

Xray: Demonstrated on plain films of pelvis or on TRUS of the prostate. May not be identified on cystoscopy

Rx: If asx, no rx necessary. If pt has sx, rx incl TURP or suprapubic prostatectomy. In the setting of multiple symptomatic prostatic calculi and intractable infections, total prostatectomy and bilateral seminal vesiculectomy are usually curative (Campbell's Urology 1992;6:2085–2156)

7 Diseases of the Penis

7.1 BALANOPOSTHITIS

Cause: Inflammation of foreskin and glans penis. May be bacterial (Ped Dermatol 1994;11:168), intertrigo, irritant dermatitis, maceration injury, or candidal in etiology (Genitourin Med 1994;70:345; 1993;69:400)

Epidem: Occurs in uncircumcised males. May be seen in children and adults. Most often occurs in males with poorly retractile foreskin

Si/Sx: Redness, edema, discharge, pain, may be assoc with voiding difficulties

Lab: KOH prep; Tzanck prep; fungal, bacterial, or viral cultures as dictated by clinical examination

DiffDx: Neoplasm, psoriasis, Zoon's balanitis, papillomavirus, other sexually transmitted diseases (Genitourin Med 1994;70:175)

Rx: Eliminate irritants, improve personal hygiene, topical antifungals if fungal related, short course of low-potency topical steroids, retraction of foreskin to allow glans and prepuce to dry after cleansing, circumcision if recurrent

7.2 LICHEN SCLEROSIS

Cause: Chronic dermatitis that may be related to abnl regulation of interleukin-1 (Hum Genet 1994;94:407)

Epidem: Occurs commonly on genital skin. Females > males. In males more common in older males (J Am Acad Dermatol 1992;26:951), may occur in children. High prevalence of autoimmune disease

Pathophys: Lesions well circumscribed white macules or plaques. Epidermis often atrophic and prone to ulceration. More common on moist skin of foreskin and in females in the vulva and perianal area. May lead to scar formation and destruction and contraction of foreskin, clitoral prepuce, and vulva

Cmplc: BXO is late stage in males

Si/Sx: May be asx, but often assoc with itching and burning. Males may note pain with urination or erection

DiffDx: Vitiligo, postinflammatory hypopigmentation, scar

Lab: Dx often made by physical examination. If question, bx is helpful

Rx: In males rx is circumcision. In females high-potency topical steroids are effective (J Reprod Med 1993;39:25)

7.3 FIXED DRUG ERUPTION

Cause: Cutaneous eruption that can be reproduced at the same site(s) by the same drug(s) (J Peds 1999;135:396)

Epidem: Medications most likely to cause reaction are oral contraceptives, barbiturates, phenolphthalein, tetracycline, salicylates, NSAIDs (Int J Dermatol 1991;30:867)

Pathophys: T-cell independent ag-specific triggering of mast cells or keratinocyte cytokine release (TNF-alpha, IL-2, IL-6) after administration of causative drug (Dermatology 1995;191:185)

Sx: May be painful

Si: Genital lesions usually solitary, well-demarcated inflammatory, may be erosive. Shaft and glans of penis are common sites. Recurrent with repeat medication exposure at same site; postinflammatory hyperpigmentation common in recurrent lesions

Lab: Bx: Papillary–dermal mononuclear cell infiltrate near dermoepidermal junction

Rx: D/c offending medication; topical care

7.4 ZOON'S BALANITIS

Cause: Plasma-cell mediated
Epidem: Uncircumcised males only. Lesions found on glans or prepuce
Pathophys: Histopathol: Band of plasma cells in dermis; may be chronic
Sx: Usually asx
Si: Solitary, red distinct borders, may be erosive, up to 2 cm in size
(Urol Int 1993;50:182)
DiffDx: Squamous cell carcinoma in situ, other forms of balanitis
Lab: Bx helpful to confirm dx
Rx: Circumcision; not always successful

7.5 BEHÇET'S SYNDROME

Nejm 1990;322:326; 1979;301:431; Bull Rheum Dis 1979;29:972
Cause: Vasculitis
Epidem: Genetic? Assoc (27%) with HLA B5 and 27; viral ? though
isolated occurrence argues against it. Male:female 1.7:1 in eastern
Mediterranean type, 1:2 U.S. in Mayo Clinic
Pathophys: Immune complex with small vessel vasculitis
Sx: Onset in 20s
Si: Recurrent: Oral ulceration primary criterion for illness. Ulcerations
either aphthous type, deep, painful, numerous, may scar; or
herpetic type, especially in females, 1–2 mm, will respond to
tetracycline oral rinse rx. Recurrent, painful. Painful genital ulcers
occur in majority of people, which is 1 of 4 secondary criteria for
dx (J Am Acad Dermatol 1995;32:968); does not always occur
concurrently with oral lesions; may involve scrotum, prepuce or
glans; may be herpetiform, major (>1 cm), or minor. Uveitis
Crs: Each attack lasts 1–4 wk. CNS disease has bad prognosis
Cmplc: Blindness (Bull Rheum Dis 1985;35:1) (rx often titrated
to the uveitis); multiple cardiac (Ann IM 1983;98:639);
inflammatory arthritis with polys >200,000; aseptic meningitis;
thrombophlebitis; colitis; skin pustules and "delayed
hypersensitivity rxn" to saline or any shot
DiffDx: Aphthous ulcers, syphilis, herpes simplex, chancroid

Lab: Heme: ESR elevated. Serol: Increased acute phase reactants. Skin tests: (+) Delayed hypersensitivity reaction to a saline shot is diagnostic

Rx: Rx of genital lesions is both local and systemic. Local: Moisture-retaining dressings, intralesional injection of corticosteroids, topical anesthetics. Systemic: (1) ASA, indomethacin, or pentoxifylline (Trental) 300 mg po bid (Ann IM 1996;124:891); (2) high-dose steroids; (3) azathioprine (Nejm 1990;322:281), cyclophosphamide, or chlorambucil; (4) thalidomide 100 mg po qd (Ann IM 1998;128:443); cmplc: teratogenicity in pregnant female, polyneuropathy. Other therapies include colchicine, FK 506, hydroxycloroquinine (Plaquenil) (J Ocul Pharmacol 1994;10:553; Curr Opin Rheumatol 1994;6:39)

7.6 SCLEROSING LYMPHANGITIS

Cause: Local trauma

Epidem: Males 20–40 yr (BJU 1987;59:194). Assoc with vigorous sexual activity (Br J Vener Dis 1972;48:545)

Pathophys: Thrombosed lymphatic vessels

Sx: Usually painless

Si: Translucent, flesh/red-colored lesion on shaft/glans of penis (Arch Dermatol 1993;129:366; Cutis 1991;47:421). Swelling proximal and parallel to the corona (J Urol 1982;127:987)

Crs: Usually remits within 4–6 wk (BJU 1987;59:194)

Rx: Avoidance of vigorous sexual activity. If persists, excise (J Urol 1982;127:987)

7.7 ERYTHEMA MULTIFORME

Cause: Many drugs (sulfonamides, penicillin, phenytoin, phenlybutazone) have been reported to cause erythema multiforme (J Invest Dermatol 1994;102:285; Nejm 1994;331:1272). May occur secondary to opiates, NSAIDs, IVP dye (steroids protect), thiamine, curare, dextrans, hormonal fluctuations. Assoc infectious agents incl *Mycoplasma pneumoniae*, *Histoplasma capsulatum*,

Coccidioides immitis, Yersinia enterocolitica, echovirus, Coxsackie virus, Epstein–Barr, influenza virus, herpes simplex

Epidem: Affects all cutaneous skin surfaces. Stevens–Johnson syndrome more severe form

Pathophys: With herpes infection, lesions appear 7–12 d after viral eruption

Sx: Sore throat, malaise

Si: Red iris or target lesions 1–2 cm in diameter. Stevens–Johnson syndrome: Targetoid lesions, blisters, mucosal membrane involvement. Toxic epidermal necrolysis: Sloughing of the epidermis and blistering

Crs: Usually resolves over 3–6 wk, but may be recurrent

Cmplc: Epidermal detachment of mucous membranes, locally in Stevens–Johnson syndrome with 5% mortality, or extensively in toxic epidermal necrolysis with 30% mortality (Nejm 1995;333:1660)

DiffDx: R/o systemic diseases like SLE, dermatomyositis, scarlet fever

Rx: Eliminate causative agent, rx denuded skin, systemic immunosuppression controversial

7.8 TUBERCULOSIS OF THE PENIS

Cause: *Mycobacterium tuberculosis*

Epidem: Rare manifestation of TB in adults, may be primary or secondary

Pathophys: Primary TB of penis occurs after sexual contact with organism present in female genital tract or by contamination from infected clothing (J Urol 1980;124:927; BJU 1976;48:274). Rarely, may develop secondary to inoculation through an infected ejaculate

Si/Sx: Superficial ulcer of glans or solid penile nodule (J Urol 1989;141:1430)

Cmplc: Tubercular cavernositis

DiffDx: Malignant penile lesions

Lab: Bx of lesion to confirm dx

Rx: Antituberculosis chemotherapy

7.9 MOLLUSCUM CONTAGIOSUM

Cause: Virus belonging to the DNA pox family

Epidem: Worldwide incidence of 2–8%. Genitalia most commonly involved, but can affect other areas of body. Requires intimate skin–skin contact for transmission. Incubation period 2–3 mo.

Crs: Usually a self-limiting benign skin lesion (Dermatol 1994;189:65); can be more severe in immunocompromised

Sx/Si: Small, firm umbilicated skin papules, smooth and pearly or flesh colored

Rx: Excise, freeze, burn; in children, less traumatically rx with cantharidin 0.7% applied with a toothpick. Topical rx with 0.5% podophyllotoxin cream effective in up to 92% pts (Dermatology 1994;189:65). Examine sexual contacts

7.10 PEARLY PENILE PAPULES

Cause: Possibly viral origin or phylogenetic residua

Epidem: 30% of men (Cutis 1977;19:54), more frequently found in young adults and uncircumcised (J Dermatol Surg Oncol 1989;15:552)

Pathophys: Histopathol: Acralangiofibromas (Arch Dermatol 1973;108:673)

Sx: Painless

Si: 1–2 mm pink/white/yellow or transparent papules that encircle corona and are more prominent on dorsal surface (GU Med 1997;73:137)

Crs: Lesions may resolve with age

DiffDx: Condyloma acuminatum, molluscum contagiosum

Rx: Reassurance; rx not necessary; if bothersome, may remove or rx with CO_2 laser (Derm Surg 1999;25:124; J Derm Surg Oncol 1989;15:552)

7.11 MELANOMA

Cause: Cutaneous malignancy

Epidem: Melanoma of male genitalia is uncommon. May occur on shaft of penis, scrotum, or more commonly glans of penis. Tends to present late

Sx/Si: Macule or papule with irregular border. May be pigmented or not. If pigmented, may be blue, red, black, or brown

Lab: Bx

Rx: Determined by depth of lesion. In general, poor prognosis with penile lesions (Eur J Surg Oncol 1997;23:277)

7.12 BASAL CELL CARCINOMA

Cause: Malignant neoplasm

Epidem: Involvement of male genitalia uncommon but may occur on penis (J Urol 1994;152:1557) or scrotum (J Am Acad Dermatol 1992;26:574)

Pathophys: Lesions occur on sun-exposed areas of those with light complexions

Sx: Often asx

Si: Papular lesion, pearly colored with telangiectasias; often ulcerate

Lab: Excisional bx confirms dx

Rx: Local excision

7.13 EXTRAMAMMARY PAGET'S DISEASE OF GENITALIA

Cause: Malignant intraepidermal process

Epidem: Females > males. Up to 80% of those with extramammary Paget's have subjacent or visceral malignancy (Cancer 1989;63:970; J Urol 1984;132:137), most commonly of urethra, bladder, rectum, sweat glands. Penile disease occurs rarely when treated with XRT for bladder cancer (BJU 1997;80:673). Affects vulva

Pathophys: Histopathol: Large, clear, vacuolated Paget cells with signs of glandular differentiation (Urology 1997;50:789). Occurs in apocrine and eccrine gland-bearing areas (BJU 1996;77:749)

Sx: Pruritic erthyematous plaque with well-demarcated borders

Si: May be excoriated and crusted

DiffDx: Bowen's disease, erythroplasia of Queyrat, melanoma, benign eczematous lesions

Lab: Bx to confirm dx; r/o underlying malignancy

Rx: Remove plaque and rx underlying malignancy. XRT and 5-FU have been used to rx plaque (Clin Oncol 1991;3:3; Tex Med 1991;87:77). Poor prognosis if invasive or mets to nodes (BJU 1996;77:749). Nd:Yag has been used for extensive extramammary Paget's disease of penis and scrotum (J d'Urol 1993;99:269)

7.14 SQUAMOUS CELL CARCINOMA IN SITU

Cause: Malignancy

Epidem: Exposure to sunlight, arsenic, and other carcinogens; hx of papilloma virus is implicated (Int J Cancer 1983;32:563; Cancer 1977;27:100)

Pathophys: Localized to epidermis. Lesions of keratinizing skin are called Bowen's disease, whereas those of mucosal surface are called erythroplasia of Queyrat

Sx: Pruritis, pain

Si: Solitary, slow-growing lesion 1–10 cm

DiffDx: Invasive squamous cell carcinoma of penis, benign papulosquamous lesion

Lab: Bx to confirm dx

Rx: Options include cryotherapy, topical vesicants, laser destruction, and surgical excision or Moh's surgery (J Urol 1994;151:829). Due to risk of invasive disease some believe excision with 5-mm margin is best rx (Urol Clin North Am 1992;19:283)

7.15 VERRUCOUS CARCINOMA

Cause: Malignancy, variant of squamous cell carcinoma
Epidem: May account for up to 24% of penile tumors (J Am Acad Dermatol 1995;32:1). Often assoc with "warty" changes. Has been assoc with nononcogenic 6 and 11 serotypes of human papillomavirus (J Am Acad Dermatol 1995;32:1). More commonly involves glans
Sx/Si: Slow-growing fungating lesion
DiffDx: Invasive squamous cell carcinoma, condyloma acuminatum
Rx: Local excision or XRT (J Urol 1995;152:1476)

7.16 PENILE CANCER

Cause: Presence of the foreskin combined with phimosis and poor personal hygiene are the most common predisposing factors (Cancer 1985;55:1618; J Urol 1976;116:458). Human papillomavirus (HPV) types 16, 18, and 33 also assoc with penile cancer (Nejm 1987;317:916; Int J Cancer 1986;37:853)
Epidem: Rare in U.S., highest incidence is in South America, India, Africa. Phimosis present in more than 50% of males with penile cancer
Pathophys: Squamous cell carcinoma accounts for 95%. Staging is by TNM classification, which follows. Primary tumor (T):
Tx Primary tumor cannot be assessed
T0 No evidence of primary tumor
Tis Carcinoma in situ
Ta Noninvasive verrucous carcinoma
T1 Tumor invades subepithelial connective tissue
T2 Tumor invades spongiosum or cavernosum
T3 Tumor invades urethra or prostate
T4 Tumor invades adjacent structure
Regional lymph nodes (N):
Nx Regional lymph nodes cannot be assessed
N0 No regional lymph node mets
N1 Mets in a single superficial inguinal lypmph node
N2 Mets in multiple or bilateral superficial inguinal lymph nodes

N3 Mets in deep inguinal or pelvic lymph node(s), unilateral or bilateral

Distant mets (M):

Mx Presence of distant mets cannot be assessed

M0 No distant mets

M1 Distant mets

(Adapted from Union Internationale Contre le Cancer. TNM Atlas: Illustrated Guide to the TNM/pTNM-Classification of Malignant Tumors, 3rd ed. New York: Springer-Verlag, 1989:237–244; and American Joint Committee on Cancer. Manual Staging for Cancer, 3rd ed. Philadelphia: Lippincott, 1988:189–191)

Sx: Often asx unless infected, which may cause pain to develop

Si: Area of induration, erythema, warty growth, nodule, or superficial elevation on the penis. 70% of lesions found on glans or prepuce. May bleed if ulcerated. If infected, may have purulent drainage. Palpable inguinal adenopathy present in 40–50% on presentation (Cancer 1993;32:1256; J Urol 1964;91:166)

Crs: If untreated may lead to complete destruction of the penis and autoamputation

Cmplc: Urinary retention and fistula formation

DiffDx: Erythroplasia of Queyrat (carcinoma in situ of the glans or foreskin), Bowen's disease (carcinoma in situ of the shaft of the penis), verrucous carcinoma, condyloma acuminatum

Lab: CBC, UA, c + s

Xray: CT scan helpful in assessing inguinal lymph nodes in obese pts and those with prior inguinal surgery. May identify pelvic adenopathy

Rx: Varies with location and size of tumor. Noninvasive small tumors of prepuce may be treated with circumcision, with a recurrence rate of 30% (Cancer 1982;49:2185; J Urol 1972;107:273, Proc R Soc Med 1975;68:781). Distal penile lesions <2–3 cm involving proximal prepuce, superficial glans, or coronal sulcus are candidates for Moh's micrographic surgery, with excellent cure rate for lesions <1 cm and 50% for lesions >3 cm (J Urol 1985;133:961). Superficial lesions may also be treated with the Nd:Yag laser or the CO_2 laser

Lesions near coronal sulcus or those involving distal glans and shaft are best treated with partial penectomy if a tumor-free margin of 2 cm can be achieved with a remaining penile length of ≥3 cm. Lesions involving proximal penile shaft or bulky lesions and those where tumor-free margins of 2 cm cannot be achieved or a short penile stump will remain are best treated by total penectomy and perineal urethrostomy

Pts with palpable lymphadenopathy 3–6 wk after rx of primary lesion and use of abx rx should undergo inguinal lymph node dissection. Use of prophylactic lymphadenectomy in the setting of nonpalpable lymph nodes is controversial. Modified lymph node dissections have decreased morbidity assoc with inguinal lymph node dissection (J Urol 1988;140:306)

7.17 KAPOSI'S SARCOMA

Cause: Human herpes-8-virus (HHV-8) coinfection (Nejm 1998;338:948; 1997;336:163; 1996;334:1168, Jama 1997;277:478)

Epidem: HHV-8 is venereally spread at least among homosexual males. Most common malignancy in AIDS pts (Nejm 1995;332:1181) with a lifetime risk of 50%. 3% of men with AIDS and Kaposi's sarcoma may initially present with a genital lesion (J Urol 1989;142:1475)

Pathophys: Endothelial-derived tumor. Histology: Proliferation of abnormal vascular structures

Sx/Si: Subcutaneous, nontender, nonpruritic nodules. Lesions may be red or blue, may become exophytic and bleed. Lymphedema may occur. Lower extremities commonly involved and may lead to penile and scrotal edema. May have fever, weight loss, night sweats—assoc with poorer prognosis

Crs: Variable. Some pts have spontaneous remissions or long intervals without disease progression

Lab: Bx may confirm dx if physical examination not definitive

Rx: Intralesional hCG (Nejm 1996;335:1261); interferon helps 50% (Nejm 1983;308:1071): Vinblastine 4–8 mg iv q1 wk (Ann IM 1985;103:335). XRT for symptomatic local disease. Laser rx, cryosurgery, and electrocoagulation also have been used

7.18 PENILE FRACTURE

Urology 1999;54:352; BJU 1996;77:279

Cause: Buckling injury to the erect penis

Epidem: Trauma to the erect penis. Usually occurs during intercourse (Urology 1999;54:352)

Pathophys: Tear of tunica albuginea that surrounds the corpora cavernosa. Male will often hear a "snap" followed by penile detumescence and penile ecchymosis

Sx: Penile pain, impotence

Si: Penile ecchymosis, penile curvature, palpable penile scar, blood at urethral meatus

Cmplc: Impotence, penile curvature, urethral disruption

Lab: Xray: Urethrography if urethral injury is suspected; MRI (Radiographics 2000;20:1397)

Rx: Immediate surgical exploration and closure of the tunica albuginea (Urology 1999;5492:352). Increased risk of complications with delayed repair (J Urol 1996;155:148)

7.19 PENILE AMPUTATION

Cause: Accidental, self-inflicted, or result of an attack (Arch Gen Psych 1979;36:441)

Epidem: Uncommon

Pathophys: Amputated segment should be placed in sterile bag containing sterile saline and placed on ice for transport. If significant bleeding, tourniquet may be applied to base of penis

Cmplc: Erectile dysfunction, sensory loss, sloughing of distal penis requiring additional penile reconstruction

Rx: Microsurgical repair of dorsal penile arteries, vein, and nerves; approximation of corpora cavernosa, debridement of devitalized and contaminated penile shaft skin, split-thickness skin grafting for skin loss (Urol Clin North Am 1989;16:359)

7.20 PENILE STRANGULATION

Cause: May be self-induced during self-mutilation or masturbation or accidental from hair or condom catheters applied too tightly

Epidem: May occur in infants, children, adults

Pathophys: Constriction leads to edema of penis distal to object; if persistent, deep trauma to penis may occur

Sx: Penile pain, voiding troubles

Si: Penile edema distal to lesion

Cmplc: Priapism, ischemia, urethral injury

Rx: Apply soap and water to penis to help remove object or apply a string starting at meatus and wrapping around glans circumferentially to compress distal penile edema and facilitate removal of object (J Urol 1993;149:372)

7.21 PRIAPISM

J Urol 1986;136:104; AUA Update 1988;29:226; Emerg Med Clin North Am 1998;6:509

Cause: Persistent erection arising from dysfunction of the mechanisms that regulate penile detumescence and flaccidity or alteration in the regulation of arterial inflow. Peak incidence ages 5–10 yr and 20–50 yr

Epidem: 30% of cases are idiopathic, 21% involve alcohol abuse or drug therapy, 12% related to perineal trauma, and 11% related to SS disease (BJU 1986;58:113). Other causes incl neurogenic factors, infections, toxins, local stimuli, inflammatory disease, malignancy, TPN, and hematologic abnl. In younger pts, priapism most often assoc with SS disease or neoplasm (BJU 1989;64:541)

Pathophys: Exact mechanism of priapism is unclear. Priapism may be divided into 2 groups: low-flow and high-flow priapism. Low-flow priapism is assoc with ischemia, veno-occlusion, and stasis of blood, which results in a rigid painful erection. May be related to excessive veno-occlusive mechanism, increased release of neurotransmitters, prolonged relaxation of cavernous smooth muscles, which raises intracavernous pressure to 80 to 120 mmHg. High-flow priapism assoc with trauma and is nonischemic and painless. Penis is not fully rigid with high-flow priapism. High-flow priapism is the result of unregulated arterial inflow

Sx: Penile pain, dysuria

Si: Fever, sepsis, urinary retention, penile swelling

Crs: After 12 h of priapism there is trabecular interstitial edema. At 24 h there is destruction of the sinusoidal endothelium and platelet aggregation. At 48 h there are thrombi in the sinusoidal spaces, smooth muscle necrosis, and corporal septal thickening (J Urol 1986;135:142)

Cmplc: Ischemia, loss of erectile function

Lab: Penile blood gas, monitoring of intracavernosal pressure. With ischemic, low-flow priapism the penile blood gas demonstrates a $pO_2 < 30$, $pCO_2 > 60$, pH < 7.25, and intracavernous pressure >40 mmHg. In high-flow priapism, penile blood gas will be nl. In patient with SS disease/trait, a hemoglobin S should be checked

Xray: Color flow Doppler sonography if high flow is suspected (pelvic/perineal trauma and/or nonischemic blood gas)

Rx: Rx varies with cause and duration of priapism. During therapy helpful to monitor intracavernous pressure. If it remains <40 mmHg for 10 min, priapism is resolved

Sickle-Cell Related: Hydrate, alkalinize, control pain, hypertransfuse, or exchange transfuse to decrease hemoglobin S to 30–40% (J Urol 1999;145:65). If priapism persists, intracavernous injection therapy should be attempted before surgical intervention

High-Flow Priapism: Intracavernous injection therapy may be attempted but often yields unsustained detumescence. Injection of methylene blue (inhibitor of cGMP phosphodiesterase and blocks effect of nitric oxide on smooth muscle) has been used successfully (J Urol 1991;146:1361). If priapism persists, perform angiography and embolization of feeding vessel

Leukemic: Conservative rx with pain medications. Local irradiation and chemotherapy may be employed if symptoms are severe

Idiopathic and Intracavernous Injection-Related: Corporal aspiration and injection of alpha-adrenergic agent (J Urol 1995;153:1182). If priapism is less than 14 h duration, injection of apha-adrenergic agent is successful in most cases (J Urol 1991;146:323). If alpha-adrenergic therapy fails, creation of Winter shunt (shunt between glans penis and coropora cavernosa) is indicated. Failures of the Winter shunt are treated with more complex shunting procedures

Apha-Adrenergic Injection for Priapism: Intermittent injection of 100–500 µg of phenylephrine every 5 min until detumescence or a maximum of 10 doses is reached. Phenylephrine is supplied as 10 mg/mL (1%) in a 1-mL vial and must be diluted with 0.9% NaCl to achieve appropriate concentration (J Urol 1995;153:1182)

7.22 ERECTILE DYSFUNCTION (ED)

Nejm 2000;342:1802.

Cause: Manifestation of disease processes or treatments that may affect the nerves, arteries, or veins involved in the erectile process. Causes include psychogenic, neurogenic (spinal cord injury, Parkinson's disease, CVA, brain tumor, Alzheimer's disease, trauma, spinal cord abnl such as myelomeningocele, MS, disk herniation), postsurgical nerve injury (APR, low anterior resection, RRPX, radical cystectomy), vitamin deficiency, alcoholism, endocrinologic (hypothalamic–pituitary dysfunction), vascular and CV, medication induced (antidepressants, antihypertensive, hormonal agents), Peyronie's disease, recreational drug abuse, and metabolic disorders (DM, hemochromatosis, SS disease, hepatic/renal failure, scleroderma, thyroid disease, adrenal disease) (Carson C, Kirby R, Goldstein I. Textbook of Erectile Dysfunction. Oxford: ISIS Medical Media, 1999)

Epidem: Affects 50% of men ages 40–70 (J Urol 1994;151:54). Higher probability of ED directly related to CV disease, HT, DM, assoc meds, and index of anger and depression. Smoking and hyperlipidemia also risk factors

Pathophys: Consistent inability to achieve and/or maintain an erection satisfactory for completion of sexual performance (NIH consensus panel). Must be distinguished from other forms of sexual dysfunction incl decreased libido and orgasmic and ejaculatory dysfunction. Erectile function is a neurovascular event. With stimulation, there is the release of nitric oxide from nonadrenergic noncholinergic neurons, which increases production of cGMP, which stimulates relaxation of cavernous smooth muscle, leading to increased blood flow to penis. As cavernosal sinusoids distend with blood, there is passive compression of subtunical veins, which decreases venous outflow. Alterations in any of these events may lead to ED

Sx: Inadequate penile rigidity or duration of rigidity, claudication, angina

Si: Signs of assoc conditions, incl palpable penile plaques, penile curvature with erection, decreased peripheral pulses, neurologic deficits, gynecomastia

Crs: If untreated, may remain the same or progress in severity

Cmplc: Loss of self-esteem, depression, relationship problems, adverse affects on quality of life

DiffDx: Decreased libido, anorgasmia, ejaculatory dysfunction

Lab: Evaluation directed at identifying underlying medical condition(s). Serum chemistries, renal function tests, CBC, UA, hormonal evaluation (testosterone and prolactin) indicated. In select cases, cholesterol, thyroid function tests and liver function tests are indicated

Xray: Duplex US with intracavernous injection (prostaglandin E1, alprostadil) 10 µg is a useful test to evaluate arterial insufficiency and veno-occlusive disease. Peak systolic velocity of <25 mL/sec indicates arterial disease (Radiology 1985;155:777). Persistent elevated diastolic flow >5–10 cm/sec suggests veno-occlusive dysfunction (Am J Radiol 1989;153:1133; Am J Radiol 1989;153:1149). Gold standard for dx and localization of arterial disease is pudendal arteriography with pharmacologic therapy (alprostadil). Gold standard for evaluation of veno-occlusive dysfunction is pharmacologic cavernosometry and cavernosography

Rx: Various rx options are available (Table 7–1). Other forms of intracavernous injection therapy (various combinations of papaverine, phentolamine, and prostaglandin E1) exist but are more difficult to obtain than prostaglandin E1 alone. Topical prostaglandin is being investigated. In select pts with arterial disease or veno-occlusive dysfunction, surgical correction may be indicated. Long-term success rates for rx of discrete arterial lesions or veno-occlusive disease in well-selected individuals are 40–60% (J Urol 1995;153:369; 1994;152:888; 1993;149:306; Int J Impot Res 1993;5:47)

Table 7-1. Treatment Options for Erectile Dysfunction

Rx	Administration	Dosing	Success Rate	Contraindications	Side Effects	Mechanisms of Action
Sildenafil (Viagra)	Oral: Taken on demand 0.5–1.5 h before intercourse, requires stimulation	25, 50, 100 mg, lower dose if >65 yr, use newer protease inhibitors, erythromycin, ketoconazole with hepatic/renal failure; 78% pts prefer 100 mg. Use only once per 24 h	48–81%; varies with etiology of erectile dysfunction	Concomitant nitrate use, retinitis pigmentosa. Relative contraindications: significant CHF, HT requiring multidrug rx	HA in 16%, flushing in 10%, dyspepsia in 7%, visual disturbance in 3%, priapism uncommon	Phosphodiesterase type V inhibitor leads to increased cGMP, which stimulates cavernous sm. muscle relaxation
Intraurethral alprostadil (MUSE)	Small suppository placed into distal urethra via small applicator	125, 250, 500, 1000 μg. Use only once per 24 h	30–66% success rate (Nejm 1997;336:1)	Hypersensitivity to PGE1, pregnant partner, predisposition to priapism (leukemia, multiple myeloma, sickle cell)	Pain (penile, urethral, testicular, perineal) in 33%, lowers blood press in 3%, priapism in 3%, vaginal irritation in 10%	Absorbed through urethral mucosa and stimulates arterial dilation and flow
Intracavernous injection therapy withprostaglandin E1 (PGE1) (Caverjet, Edex)	Direct injection into lateral aspect of corpora cavernosa, alternating sides with each injection	5 μg to >40 μg; dose depends on etiology of ED; test dose at 10 μg; if suspect neurologic disease, use 5-μg test dose; use only once per 48–72 h	Average success rate 73% (Int J Impot Res 1994;6:149; J Urol 1988;140:66)	Known hypersensitivity to alprostadil. Pts at risk for priapism: Pts at increased risk: those on anticoagulants and with Peyronie's dz	Prolonged erections in 1.1–1.3%, corporal fibrosis in 2.7%, painful erection in 15–30%, hematoma, ecchymosis in 1.5%	PGE1 stimulates cavernous sm. muscle relaxation, causes modulation of adenyl cyclase, increase in cAMP and subsequent free Ca^{2+} conc

Table 7–1. (*cont'd*)

Rx	Administration	Dosing	Success Rate	Contraindications	Side Effects	Mechanisms of Action
Vacuum constriction device	Plastic cylinder with hand or battery-operated pump and constricting bands	N/A. Remove band within 30 min after application	68–83% satisfaction rate	Painful ejaculation: 3–16%, inability to ejaculate: 12–30%, petechiae of penis: 25–39%, numbness during erection: 5% (J Urol 1993;149:290; *Textbook of Erectile Dysfunction*)	Use with caution in pts taking aspirin or anticoagulants	Vacuum device creates negative pressure that "pulls" blood into corpora cavernosa; constriction band prolongs erection by decreasing corporal venous drainage
Penile prosthesis	Surgically placed, models range from semirigid to inflatable	N/A	>90% satisfaction with inflatable prostheses (J Urol 1993;150:1814; 1992;147:62)	*Decreases penile length by 1 cm.* Infection <10%, diabetics at increased risk. Mechanical malfunction <5% (Urol Clin North Am 1995;22:847). Erosion: increased risk in diabetics and spinal cord injury pts	Requires counseling, preoperative	Cylinders placed in corpora cavernosa provide penile rigidity; once placed, there is corporal fibrosis; if removed, remaining options less likely to work

7.23 PEYRONIE'S DISEASE

Cause: Exact etiology unknown. It appears that trauma to tunica albuginea and surrounding tissue leads to plaque (scar) formation in certain people

Epidem: Identified in 1% of white males. Highest incidence is in age group 45–60 yr (BJU 1982;54:748). 16–20% have assoc Dupuytren's contractures (BJU 1982;54:748; J Bone Joint Surg (UK) 1963;45:709). Peyronie's couples often participate in frequent and vigorous intercourse and employ positions traumatic to the penis. Two subsets: those who experience an insidious onset of sx and those who have an acute onset with little or no progression of the disease

Pathophys: Plaques are located in the midline on dorsal or ventral surface and may extend laterally to involve adjacent areas of tunica albuginea. Buckling injury during intercourse or trauma leads to intravasation of blood and resulting inflammation, induration and scarring of tunica albuginea in susceptible individuals (J Urol 1997;157:311)

Sx: ≥1/3 will have painful erections, 19–20% with ED (J Urol 1975;114:69)

Si: Palpable penile plaque, during erection the penis deviates toward the plaque

Cx: Penile pain, ED, penile curvature

DiffDx: Penile fracture, congenital chordee

Xray: May identify calcification within the plaque on penile US or plain film

Rx: Reassurance. Peyronie's disease is an evolving process; in some pts it can resolve or improve significantly and no surgical rx is necessary. Initial rx is medical with vitamin E 400 mg po bid (Prog Reprod Biol 1983;9:41). Vitamin E is a free-radical scavenger. Other medical therapies: Para-aminobenzoic acid (PABA) 12 gm/d (24 500-mg tabs or 6 2-gm packets), but is expensive and has GI side effects (Techniques Urol 1997;3:135). If erections painful, try fexofenadine (Allegra) 60 mg po bid for 3 mo. Colchicine (0.6 mg po bid) for 2–3 wk then check CBC; if no bone marrow suppression, continuing for 3–4 mo has been anecdotally shown to be helpful. It may lower sperm count and have GI side effects. Other rxs: Intralesional rxs such as verapamil

(J Urol 1997;158:1395) and XRT. When the disease has stabilized and there is persistent disabling penile curvature and or ED, surgical rx is indicated. Erectile function should first be assessed with Doppler studies after pharmacologically induced erection. Depending on erectile function, surgical options incl contralateral plication of tunica albuginea (may cause penile shortening) (Urol Clin North Am 1989;16:607), plaque excision and grafting (J Urol 1974;111:44), or penile prosthesis with/without penile moulding (J Urol 1994;152:1121)

7.24 HEMOSPERMIA

Cause: Blood in ejaculate may be assoc with pathology of prostate, seminal vesicles, or urethra; infection; secondary to trauma; or related to systemic diseases (Urology 1995;46:463)

Epidem: Prevalence unknown, although hemospermia common

Pathophys: Prostatic pathology assoc with hemospermia includes polyps, vascular lesions, calculi, inflammatory disorders, and malignancy. Bladder and urethral lesions include tumors, urethritis, urethral polyps, utricular cyst, urethral stricture, and urethral condyloma. Lesions of seminal vesicles include cysts, carcinoma, calculi, and infections. Systemic disorders include HT, bleeding disorders, and lymphoma (Urology 1995;46:463)

Sx: Sx may be referable to the underlying etiology

Si: Blood in ejaculate. Check blood pressure to rule out HT

Crs: Often self-limiting and related to benign pathology

DiffDx: Melanospermia and hematuria

Lab: UA, c + s, PSA, urethral swabs for gc and chlamydia, semen analysis, clotting studies if bleeding disorder is suspected

Xray: Transrectal US indicated for chronic hemospermia. MRI may be helpful to visualize seminal vesicle pathology

Other: Cystoscopy indicated for chronic hemospermia

Rx: Reassurance is best, as condition is related to benign disease in most cases. If infectious, treat with abx. Urethral or prostatic varices can be fulgurated. Aspiration of seminal vesicle cysts, rx of bleeding disorders

Section II

PEDIATRIC UROLOGY

Section II

PEDIATRIC UROLOGY

8 Diseases of the Kidney and Ureter in Children

8.1 RENAL AGENESIS

Cause: Embryologic anomaly that appears related to developmental anomaly of ureteric bud (Development 1996;122:1919). May also be related to regression of MCDK (J Urol 1993;150:793) (see 8.4).

Epidem: Bilateral renal agenesis is rare and occurs in 1 of 4000 births. Unilateral renal agenesis occurs in 1 of 1000–1500 (Am J Dis Child 1974;127:17; Mayo Clin Proc 1966;41:538). Males > females

Pathophys: For nl renal development, a nl ureteral bud must penetrate a nl metanephric blastema. Assoc genital anomalies occur more often in females and include uterus didelphys and vaginal agenesis. In males, hypospadias, UDTs, vasal anomalies, and cysts of the seminal vesicle and prostate have been noted (Int Urol Nephrol 1988;20:29). Other assoc anomalies include chromosomal syndromes and cardiac, skeletal, GI, respiratory anomalies (Obstet Gynecol 1997;90:26; Ped Nephrol 1996;10:498; Adv Ped 1995;42:575; J Med Genet 1995;21:153; Am J Dis Child 1974;127:17). GU anomalies seen in up to 48% and include VUR (28%), UVJ obstruction (11%), UPJO (7%) (J Urol 1999;162:1081)

Sx: Asx if unilateral. If bilateral, virtually fatal from respiratory compromise

Si: Ipsilateral nonpalpable vas deferens and other assoc genital anomalies

Crs: Renal failure and respiratory distress if lesion is bilateral. With unilateral renal agenesis, may be at increased risk of proteinuria,

HT, and renal insufficiency in the long term (Ped Nephrol 1992;6:412)

Cmplc: See above

DiffDx: Ectopic kidney (see 8.2) and involuted MCDK

Lab: UA

Xray: IVP or DMSA scan to rule out ectopic kidney and VCUG to r/o contralateral VUR

Rx: Rx of assoc congenital anomalies. With unilateral agenesis, follow-up of blood pressure, UA, and renal function indicated over the long term

8.2 ECTOPIC KIDNEY

Cause: Failure of kidney to reach normal location

Epidem: Incidence: 1 in 900 (Urol Int 1959;9:63); L > R; may be ectopic to pelvic, iliac, abdominal, thoracic, contralateral, or crossed locations. Bilateral in 10% (Mayo Clin Proc 1971;46:461). 90% of crossed ectopic kidneys are fused to ipsilateral kidney; solitary crossed ectopia usually involves L kidney migrating to R side with absence of R kidney. Males > females

Pathophys: Ureter enters into normal side of the bladder

Crs: Increased incidence of hydronephrosis and calculi (J Urol 1994;151:1660). May be at increased risk for injury from blunt trauma

Cmplc: Assoc anomalies: Contralateral agenesis, contralateral hydronephrosis secondary to VUR or obstruction in up to 25% (J Urol 1994;151:1660); genital anomalies in up to 45% (Urology 1973;1:51); skeletal anomalies in 50% with solitary crossed renal ectopia and 40% with genital anomalies (Urology 1991;38:556). Rarely, adrenal gland absent or abnormally located

Si/Sx: Asx; if obstructed may have pain atypical for renal colic

Xray: May be identified on IVP, renal US, radionuclide scanning, or retrograde pyelography

Rx: Not necessary unless obstruction or calculus

8.3 HORSESHOE KIDNEY

Cause: Renal fusion abnormality

Epidem: Incidence: 1 in 400 (Nejm 1959;261:684). Male:female 2:1; 95% of cases kidneys join at lower pole (Clin Radiol 1975;26:409). Seen in 20% pts with trisomy 18 and up to 60% females with Turner's syndrome (Peds 1988;82:852)

Pathophys: Originates at 4–6 wk gestation. Pelves and ureters usually anteriorly located, crossing ventral to isthmus. Inferior mesenteric artery prevents complete ascent

Sx: 1/3 asx; may present with vague abdominal pain

Si: Rarely a palpable midline abdominal mass

Crs: High incidence of congenital anomalies including skeletal, CV, CNS

Cmplc: Hydronephrosis, infection, stone; increased incidence of Wilms' tumor (2×) (J Urol 1985;133:1002)

Lab: If sx, obtain UA, c + s to r/o UTI

Xray: US or IVP will demonstrate horseshoe kidney—kidneys low lying, close to vertebral column, continuity of outer border of lower pole of each kidney toward and across midline, high insertion of ureter into renal pelvis and anteriorly displaced ureter draping over midline mass (isthmus), calyces posterior to renal pelvis

Rx: No rx necessary; if stones or obstruction, rx accordingly

8.4 MULTICYSTIC DYSPLASTIC KIDNEY (MCDK)

Cause: Exact cause unknown. Proposed etiologies include atresia of the ureter or renal pelvis, which leads to severe hydronephrosis (Semin Roentgenol 1975;10:113); and failure of union of ureteric bud and metanephric blastema, which leads to cystic dilation (Arch Klin Chir 1894;48:343)

Epidem: L > R. One of most common causes of abdominal mass in infants. Contralateral UPJO found in 3–12% of infants with MCDK. Contralateral VUR seen in 18–43% of infants (J Peds 1992;121:65). More commonly identified in utero; when detected by US, may be bilateral in 19–34% of cases (Radiology 1986;161:27)

Pathophys: Ureteral and/or pelvic atresia leads to severe hydronephrosis. Also, renal vessels are small or absent. Typically kidneys have little (≤10%) or no function on functional renal scan (DMSA)

Sx: If kidney is markedly enlarged, there may be respiratory compromise. HT rarely reported

Si: Abdominal mass

Crs: Typically these kidneys will involute over time and no longer be identifiable by US. Rarely, kidney size will increase. Rare potential for malignant degeneration (Wilms' tumors, embryonal cell tumor, RCC) in MCDKs

Cmplc: HT, respiratory insufficiency, malignancy

DiffDx: UPJO

Lab: If both sides appear to be affected, test serum BUN, creatinine levels

Xray: Renal US shows collection of renal cysts of various sizes with no larger central or medial cyst. Often little if any identifiable renal parenchyma. DMSA renal scan shows little if any ipsilateral renal function. VCUG should be obtained on children with MCDKs to r/o contralateral VUR

Rx: In absence of respiratory compromise or HT, follow-up US studies indicated until kidney has completely involuted. Contralateral VUR if present should be treated according to routine management of VUR

8.5 URETEROPELVIC JUNCTION OBSTRUCTION (UPJO)

Cause: May be primary or secondary, related to intrinsic or extrinsic pathology. Exact cause of UPJO is not fully understood, but may be related to incomplete canalization of ureter during development. Histopathologic evaluation of UPJ reveals increased collagen and decreased smooth muscle. Smooth muscle is disoriented and there are more circular smooth muscle fibers than longitudinal fibers (J Urol 1976;116:725). Less common intrinsic causes include valvular mucosal folds (J Urol 1980;123:742), persistent fetal convolutions (J Urol 1979;122:251), and proximal ureteral polyps (J Urol 1981;126:796). Extrinsic obstruction may be secondary to aberrant lower pole vessels. Secondary UPJO may occur in setting of high-grade VUR (Am J Roentgenol 1983;140:231)

Epidem: Incidence is 5 cases per 100,000. Males > females (3–4:1). Occurrence sporadic, but familial tendency has been described (BJU 1985;57:365). Left kidney affected more often than the right. In 10% of cases there is coexisting VUR (Urol Clin North Am, 1998;25:173). Bilateral UPJs are diagnosed in 21–36% of cases of neonatally detected UPJOs (J Urol 1988;140:1216). Another urologic anomaly may be found in up to 50% of affected children (Radiol Clin North Am 1977;15:49)

Pathophys: Histopathologic alterations at UPJ result in inefficient propulsion of urine through UPJ and dilation of renal pelvis and calyces. Ureter may have high insertion on renal pelvis

Sx: Intermittent abdominal/flank pain in older children and adults, often asx in infants

Si: Palpable flank mass which transilluminates in children and infants, hematuria, failure to thrive, feeding difficulties, UTI, HT

Crs: If obstruction is significant and remains untreated, may lead to diminished renal function, increased risk of stone formation and infection, and renin-mediated HT

DiffDx: Obstruction due to other causes such as a retroperitoneal mass, UVJ obstruction, nonobstructive dilation

Lab: UA, c + s. If bilateral, serum BUN, creatinine

Xray: UPJO often detected during prenatal US evaluation. Hydronephrosis most common abnl detected on prenatal US evaluations and accounts for 50% of all prenatally detected lesions (Lancet 1990;336:387). Approximately 50% of cases of prenatally detected hydronephrosis will be caused by UPJO (Urol Clin North Am 1998;25:173). All children with hydronephrosis should undergo a VCUG to r/o obstruction secondary to VUR (Am J Roentgenol 1983;140:231). A Lasix Mag-3 renal scan is useful to determine renal function and degree of obstruction. Drainage response to Lasix is used to gauge degree of obstruction: if t1/2 (time needed for half the radionuclide to drain from collecting system) <10 min, there is no obstruction; if 10–20 min, it is indeterminate; if >20 min, a significant obstruction exists. Split renal functions are also calculated

Rx: Surgical intervention indicated in setting of (1) sx UPJO, (2) increasing hydronephrosis on US, (3) increasing t1/2 on Lasix Mag-3 renal scan, (4) decreasing renal function on renal scan. In pediatric population, rx of primary UPJO is routinely performed as open procedure (dismembered pyeloplasty) whereby abnl proximal ureter and redundant renal pelvis are excised and ureter anastomosed to pelvis in a dependent fashion. Pediatric secondary UPJOs (failed primary repairs) and primary and secondary UPJOs in adults may be treated via endoscopic or percutaneous approach and endopyelotomy, whereby narrowed segment is incised fully and ureter stented allowing for healing to occur around stent (J Urol 1997;158:1534;157S:244). Cmplcs of both procedures include urinary extravasation, infection, recurrent obstruction. Significant bleeding requiring open exploration has been reported with endopyelotomy

8.6 VESICOURETERAL REFLUX (VUR)

Cause: Primary VUR due to deficiency of longitudinal muscle of intravesical ureter which results in inadequate valvular mechanism. Secondary VUR occurs as result of elevated bladder pressures. Conditions assoc with increased bladder pressure incl neurogenic bladder, bladder outlet obstruction, nonneurogenic neurogenic bladder, DI

Epidem: Overall incidence in normal children is 1–18.5%. VUR identified in up to 70% of infants presenting with UTIs (J Urol 1966;95:27). Females > males, but males who present with a UTI more likely to have VUR. White girls 10 times more likely to have VUR than black girls (J Urol 1982;127:747). Siblings of pts with VUR have increased risk of VUR, and children of those with VUR are at increased risk (J Urol 1992;148:1739)

Pathophys: During elevations in bladder pressure (such as during voiding), UVJ usually occluded. This flap-valve effect accomplished by oblique entry of ureter into bladder, adequate muscular attachments to provide fixation and support, and adequate submucosal tunnel (Urol Clin North Am 1974;1:144). In primary VUR, submucosal tunnel is short in proportion to ureteral diameter. Normal submucosal tunnel is approximately 5 times diameter of ureter (J Urol 1959;82:573). Assoc abnl incl UPJO, ureteral duplication, bladder diverticula

Sx: Usually asx. If the child develops UTI, may lead to pyelonephritis and child may later present with back pain, dysuria, N/V

Si: Fever and chills may accompany a UTI. In newborns, failure to thrive may be sign of recurrent infections

Crs: Sterile VUR itself does not appear to be harmful. Pyelonephritis in a child may lead to subsequent renal scarring and HT. VUR may resolve over time. Rates of resolution vary with grade of reflux: In grades I–II, 80–85% chance of resolution (BMJ 1977;2:228; Urol Clin North Am 1974;1:144); grade III resolves in 50% of pts (J Urol 1992;148:1683; Am J Kidney 1983;3:139); and grades IV–V seldom resolve spontaneously. The younger the child at initial presentation, the more likely the VUR will resolve

Cmplc: If UTI is present, renal scarring and HT may occur

DiffDx: R/out assoc conditions such as posterior urethral valves, voiding dysfunction, and neurogenic bladder. Condition often found in such urologic disorders as bladder exstrophy, prune belly syndrome, and may be found in contralateral kidney of a pt with MCDK

Lab: UA, c + s

Xray: VUR may be identified on a contrast VCUG or radionuclide VCUG. Contrast is best initial study, as it allows for grading of reflux (Fig. 8–1), assessment of bladder capacity, PVR, and urethra. Renal US typically obtained for a baseline assessment of renal size, parenchymal thickness, and to detect hydronephrosis. DMSA scan is best for assessing renal scarring

Rx: In most cases, initial rx is medical with prophylactic abx and follow-up studies every 12–18 mo to assess VUR resolution. For infants under 8 wk, amoxicillin or ampicillin is used. For children older than 8 wk, Tm/S (Bactrim) or nitrofurantoin is used. Typical dose is 1/2 to 1/3 of usual daily dose. In older children (>10–12 yr) with lower grades of VUR and no significant scarring, may d/c prophylaxis and observe child. If recurrent UTIs occur, surgical rx indicated

Surgical rx indicated for children with high-grade VUR that fails to improve over time, breakthough UTIs, problems with complying with medical rx, persistent VUR, and VUR assoc with other anomalies such as a bladder diverticula. Surgical options include open, laparoscopic, and endoscopic procedures. Success of open procedures is 98–99% (J Urol 1992;148:359; 1991;146:352). Cmplc of surgery include infection, bleeding, obstruction, persistent reflux, and contralateral VUR

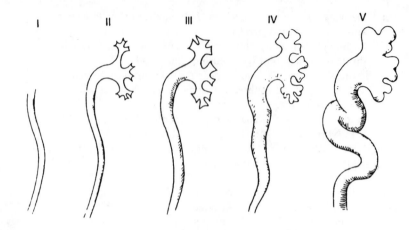

GRADES OF REFLUX

Figure 8–1. Grading of vesicoureteral reflux. (Reproduced with permission from Atala A, Keating M. Vesicoureteral reflux and megaureter. In Walsh et al., eds. Campbell's urology, 7th ed. Philadelphia: Saunders, 1998:1865.)

8.7 MEGAURETER

Cause: Megaureters are classified as primary or secondary and as refluxing, obstructive, or nonrefluxing nonobstructive (Urology 1978;11:231; Radiology 1971;99:503)

Epidem: Primary obstructed megaureter occurs 3–5 times more often in males, 2–3 times more common on the left. Bilateral in 15–25% patients (BJU 1970;42:140). Familial megaureters are rare (Urol Radiol 1981;3:185)

Pathophys: In primary obstructive megaureter there is often an area of abnl muscular development and collagen deposition in distal ureter, which affects peristalsis of distal segment (J Urol 1970;103:134). In primary refluxing megaureter, there is a congenital anomaly of UVJ (see the preceding section on VUR). Secondary obstructive megaureter occurs most often with neurogenic and non-neurogenic voiding dysfunction or obstruction (posterior urethral valves). Elevated bladder pressures (>40 cm H$_2$O) impede ability of ureter to propel urine across UVJ, leading to stasis and ureteral dilation. Same conditions may lead to secondary refluxing megaureter

Primary nonobstructive nonrefluxing megaureter usually found in newborns. May be related to transient obstruction or infant hyperreflexic bladder (J Urol 1994;152:692). Secondary nonobstructive nonrefluxing megaureter may result from UTI as a result of inhibition of ureteral peristalsis from bacterial endotoxins or from conditions assoc with high urine output (lithium toxicity, diabetes insipidus, DM, SS nephropathy, psychogenic polydipsia)

Sx: Usually asx if no obstructions or infections. If obstruction occurs, pt may experience flank pain, N/V

Si: Fever and chills if infection is present

Crs: If obstruction present, renal function may be affected

Cmplc: Increased risk of UTI

Lab: UA, c + s

Xray: Renal/bladder US assesses renal parenchyma thickness, collecting system dilation, PVR, and ureteral diameter. Contrast VCUG is obtained to determine if there is VUR and to assess bladder and urethra. Diuretic renal scan (Lasix Mag-3) helps evaluate obstruction and renal function

Rx: Rx varies with etiology. In primary refluxing megaureter, initial rx is prophylaxis during infancy and tapered ureteral reimplantation at an older age. In secondary refluxing megaureter, primary cause treated first and VUR treated second. Primary obstructive megaureter treated with prophylaxis and close observation during infancy and tapered reimplantation when the child is older (1–2 yr) as long as child is stable. Distal ureterostomy performed for infants with breakthrough infections, followed by tapered reimplantation when child is older. Nonobstructing nonrefluxing megaureters are followed conservatively. Cmplc of surgery include infection, bleeding, obstruction, persistent VUR

8.8 ECTOPIC URETER

Cause: Develops when ureteric bud has high origin from mesonephric duct with delayed or absent separation from mesonephric duct

Epidem: Incidence is estimated to be 1 in 1900, and 80% of the cases involve an upper pole ureter of a duplicated collecting system. In males, ectopic ureter usually drains a single collecting system (Eur Urol 1976;2:64; J Urol 1969;41:428). In 10% of cases, bilateral ectopic ureters occur (Br J Surg 1958;45:344). Females affected 6 times more often than males (J Urol 1972;107:308)

Pathophys: Correlation btn location of ectopic ureter and degree of renal hypoplasia or dysplasia. In setting of bilateral single system ectopic ureters, bladder neck fails to develop. Ectopic sites in the female include level of bladder neck or proximal urethra (30%), vaginal vestibule near the urethral meatus or into a Gartner's duct cyst (Am J Radiol 1970;110:540), vagina, cervix, or uterus. In males the most common ectopic site is posterior urethra (J Urol 1972;108:389). Other sites incl seminal vesicle and epididymis (Urology 1979;21:369)

Sx: Dysuria and frequency are often present with UTIs. Epididymal pain and swelling may be present in males with epididymitis (J Urol 1987;138:1100). Flank pain may be present

Si: Daytime and nighttime incontinence in females. Foul-smelling vaginal discharge may be present if ectopic to vagina. Mass on anterior vaginal wall may be a ureter ectopic to Gartner's duct cyst. Abdominal mass may be palpable. The child may present with recurrent UTIs and males may present with epididymitis

Crs: Often not detected at birth and identified during a workup for incontinence, UTI, or epididymitis

Cmplc: Recurrent UTI, incontinence, urosepsis

DiffDx: Ureterocele and UVJ obstruction

Lab: UA, c + s

Xray: Renal/bladder US may demonstrate a dysplastic/hypoplastic and/or hydronephrotic-appearing kidney, with dilated ureter visualized behind bladder (Am J Radiol 1977;129:113). IVP or CT scan may be more helpful in delineating urinary tract anatomy (Ped Clin North Am 1985;32:1353). In setting of duplicated collecting systems, a DMSA scan will aid in assessment of upper-pole function. VCUG should be obtained to r/o associated VUR

Other Eval: Vaginoscopy in females. Cystoscopy at the time of surgery in both sexes

Rx: Rx based on function of ipsilateral renal unit. If upper pole demonstrates good function, ureteropyelostomy or ureteroureterostomy can be performed. If upper pole demonstrates poor function, partial nephrectomy and ureterectomy is indicated. In a single system ectopic ureter with adequate renal function, a ureteral reimplantation is performed; if function is poor, nephroureterectomy should be performed

8.9 URETEROCELE

Cause: A cystic dilatation of the terminal ureter. Proposed etiologies incl incomplete dissolution of Chwalla's membrane, abnl detrusor musculature, and simultaneous expansion of the intravesical ureter at the time of bladder expansion (J Urol 1981;126:726; Aust NZ J Surg 1971;40:239; Urol Cutan Rev 1927;31:499)

Epidem: Ureteroceles increasingly identified on prenatal ultrasound. Female:male ratio 4:1. Occur almost exclusively in Caucasians. 10% are bilateral; 80% arise from upper pole of a duplicated collecting system. Single system ureteroceles usually found in adults. Most common presentation is UTI/urosepsis (J Urol 1995;153:166)

Pathophys: If ureterocele large enough, it can obstruct the bladder neck or contralateral ureter

Cmplc: Calculus formation (J Ped Surg 1987;22:1047), prolapse of ureterocele through urethra, hydronephrosis

DiffDx: Mesonephric duct cyst, ectopic ureter (BJU 1995;75:401)

Lab: UA, c + s to r/o UTI

Xray: Renal/bladder US often can identify a duplex kidney and dilated upper pole ureter. Thin-walled cyst (ureterocele) can often be identified in the bladder. Pitfalls of U/S: If bladder is too distended, the ureterocele may be effaced and not noted; if bladder is empty, ureterocele may not be seen. IVP: Upper pole typically functions poorly; upper pole deviated laterally from the spine due to hydronephrosis. Lower pole pushed laterally and inferiorly and lower pole ureter usually laterally deviated by dilated upper pole ureter. VCUG: Usually demonstrates size and location of ureterocele. Also notes presence/absence of VUR. VUR seen in up to 65% of lower pole ureters (BJU 1992;70:196) and in the contralateral ureter in 28% pts (J Ped Surg 1992;7:192). DMSA nuclear scan is helpful in assessing degree of upper pole function

Rx: Individual rx. Goals: (1) preservation of renal function, (2) elimination of infection, obstruction and VUR, (3) preservation of continence. Rx options include upper pole nephrectomy and partial ureterectomy, ureteropyelostomy, endoscopic incision of ureterocele, and excision of ureterocele and common sheath ureteral reimplantation. Single-system ureteroceles are often associated with a functioning renal moiety and may be treated by endoscopic incision or excision and ureteral reimplantation

8.10 CONGENITAL MESOBLASTIC NEPHROMA

Cause: Renal neoplasm. Generally benign, but mets and recurrent tumor have been reported (Cancer 1993;72:2499). Exact cause not known but tumor induction is thought to occur when multifocal blastema is primarily stromagenic (Cancer 1992;70:2358; J Urol 1981;12:513)

Epidem: Occurs predominantly in infants (most common renal tumor in infants), more commonly in children <6 mo. Rare in adults (Cancer 1982;49:573). Accounts for about 2% of childhood renal tumors. Males > females

Pathophys: Congenital mesoblastic nephroma is an infantile spindle cell tumor of the kidney. Two histologic types: cellular and classical. Cellular type is identical to congenital fibrosarcoma (Cancer Res 1998;58:5046). Chromosomal abnormalities including polysomes for chromosomes 8, 11, 17, and 20 are common. In addition, t (12:15) translocation and the assoc ETV6-NTRK3 fusion are seen (Am J Pathol 1998;153:1451). 14% of children with congenital mesoblastic nephroma have other congenital anomalies (J Ped Surg 1982;17:826)

Sx: Respiratory distress if tumor is large

Si: Polyhdramnios, abdominal mass that does not transilluminate, hematuria, perinatal anemia, and shock if mass ruptures

Crs: If untreated, may cause respiratory compromise or mets

Cmplc: Mets rarely

DiffDx: Wilms' tumor

Lab: UA, c + s, CBC if hemorrhage is suspected, ABG if respiratory distress occurs

Xray: Lesion may often be detected on prenatal US. Radiologic studies cannot reliably distinguish congenital mesoblastic nephroma from other lesions. CT scan will show a heterogeneous solid mass arising from the kidney

Rx: Stabilize newborn and then perform elective surgery. Emergency surgery is indicated if there is circulatory disturbance, respiratory distress related to the size of the lesion, and/or impending rupture is suspected (J Ped Surg 1993;28:1607). Complete excision is curative in most pts. Local recurrence may occur in pts with the cellular variant. Risk of recurrence is low in children <3 mo (Cancer 1993;72:2499). Adjuvant rx may be considered in pts with the cellular variant who have undergone incomplete resection (J Urol 1989;142:479)

8.11 WILMS' TUMOR

Urol Clin North Am 27(3):423

Cause: Malignant neoplasm

Epidem: 5–6% of all childhood cancers in U.S. (Med Pediatr Oncol 1993;21:172). 80% of GU cancers in children <15 yr (Am Cancer Soc, Atlanta, 1978). Peak incidence age 3–4 yr, 90% occurring before age 7 yr, 10% bilateral

Pathophys: ? Secondary to proliferation of metanephric blastema without nl differentiation into tubules and glomeruli (Campbell's Urology 1998;7(74):2210–2256). Loss of function of recessive tumor suppressor gene in 11p13 (WT1) region is impt (Science 1989;246:1387; Nature 1984;309:170). Also abnls of distal portion of 11p15 (WT2) seen with Wilms' tumor in Beckwith–Wiedemann syndrome (Mol Cell Biol 1989;9:1799; Hum Genet 1988;81:41). Absence of long arm of chromosome 16 in 20% of Wilms' tumors (Cancer Res 1992;52:3094). Histopath divided into favorable and unfavorable histology. Unfavorable histology: anaplastic, rhabdoid (mets to brain), clear cell sarcoma of kidney (mets to bone). Staging:

Stage I Tumor limited to kidney, completely excised, capsule intact, not ruptured, no residual tumor apparent beyond margins of resection

Stage II Tumor extends beyond kidney (regional extension, tumor in vessels outside kidney) but is completely removed, may have undergone previous bx or spillage of tumor confined to the flank, no residual tumor apparent at or beyond margins of excision

Stage III Residual nonhematogenous tumor confined to abdomen, any one of the following:
  a. Positive lymph nodes on bx in the hilus, periaortic chains, or beyond
  b. Diffuse peritoneal contamination by tumor, either via spillage beyond the flank or via tumor penetration through the peritoneal surface
  c. Peritoneal tumor implants
  d. Tumor extends beyond surgical margins, grossly or microscopically
  e. Tumor not completely resected due to local extension into vital structures

Stage IV Hematogenous mets beyond stage II such as liver, bone, brain

Stage V Bilateral renal involvement at dx. Need to stage each side (Cancer 1989;64:349)

Sx: Abdominal pain

Si: Abdominal mass, increased abdominal girth, HT, varicocele, hernia, CHF, pleural effusion.

Crs: 15% have other congenital anomalies: aniridia, hemihypertrophy, Beckwith–Wiedemann syndrome, neurofibromatosis, musculoskeletal anomalies, GU anomalies (Cancer 1976;37:403)

Cmplc: Secondary malignancies including sarcomas, adenocarcinomas, leukemias. Most sarcomas found in previous fields of XRT for the Wilms' tumor

DiffDx: Neuroblastoma, rhabdomyosarcoma, hepatoblastoma, lymphoma, lymphosarcoma, mesenteric cyst, choledochal cyst, intestinal duplication cysts, splenomegaly, hydronephrosis, MCDK, polycystic kidney, congenital mesoblastic nephroma

Lab: Serum: CBC may show polycythemia; UA, microhematuria may be present; BUN/creatinine, liver enzymes

Xray: IVP: Distortion of calyces secondary to an intrarenal mass, which may have an eggshell pattern of calcification; affected kidney may not be visualized (J Ped Surg 1988;23:152). Renal US: Heterogeneous echo pattern to tumor (Radiology 1981;140:147). Allows for visualization of renal vein and inferior vena cava to r/o intraluminal tumor (Radiology 1979;132:421). MRI allows for assessment of size and extent of tumor. C-xray or CT of chest to r/o pulmonary mets. CT of brain if rhabdoid variant

Rx: Depends on tumor histology and stage. Goal is preservation of renal function. National Wilms' Tumor Study V guidelines:

Stage I, favorable or anaplastic: Dactinomycin and vincristine

Stage II, favorable histology: Dactinomycin and vincristine

Stage III and IV, favorable: Dactinomycin, doxorubicin, vincristine, and XRT

Stage II to IV, focal anaplasia: Dactinomycin, doxorubicin, vincristine, and XRT

Stage II to IV, diffuse anaplasia: Cyclophosphamide, etoposide, vincristine, doxorubicin, XRT

Stage I to IV, clear cell sarcoma: Cyclophosphamide, etoposide, vincristine, doxorubicin, XRT

Stage I to IV, rhabdoid: Carboplatinum, etoposide, cyclophosphamide

Surgery, first look: Assess contralateral kidney, resectability, and bx lesion and any enlarged hilar or para-aortic nodes if deemed unresectable. If unilateral and resectable, resect. With bilateral disease: Bx both kidneys, sample nodes, excisional bx performed only if 2/3 of total renal parenchyma can be preserved; otherwise close and give chemo based on stage and histology of more advanced tumor and perform second look. 4-yr survival varies with stage and histology, ranging from 26% with rhabdoid sarcoma to 97% with stage I favorable histology (Cancer 1989;64:349)

9 Diseases of the Bladder in Children

9.1 BLADDER EXSTROPHY

Cause: Embryologic maldevelopment

Epidem: 3.3 cases in 100,000 live births (Tetralogy 1987;36:221). Male:female ratio 2.3:1 to 6:1 (Tetralogy 1987;36:221; J Urol 1982;127:974). Risk of recurrence of bladder exstrophy in a given family is 1 in 100 (J Med Genet 1980;17:139). Risk of bladder exstrophy in offspring of individual with bladder exstrophy and epispadias is 1 in 70 live births (J Urol 1984;132:308)

Pathophys: May occur secondary to abnl overdevelopment of cloacal membrane, preventing medial migration of mesenchymal tissue and proper lower abdominal wall development (J Urol 1964;92:659). Timing of rupture of cloacal membrane determines the variant of the exstrophy–epispadias complication that results. Other proposed etiologies exist

Cmplc: Assoc with defects of abdominal wall, genitalia, rectum, anus. Anus is displaced anteriorly. Umbilical hernia usually present. 6.7% incidence congenital vertebral malformations (BJU 1997;79:975). Inguinal hernias common. Penile abnl: Episadias (urethral meatus present on dorsal surface of penis, typically at penopubic junction), chordee, short urethral groove, shorter anterior corporal cavernosal length. Female genital anomalies: Short urethra and vagina, bifid clitoris, divergent labia and mons pubis. Vaginal orifice may be stenotic, displaced anteriorly. VUR present in nearly 100% of closed bladder exstrophies

Sx: Often asx

Si: Bladder visible on anterior abdominal wall, widened symphysis pubis, genital anomalies, inguinal hernias common

Cmplc: Wound dehiscence, small functional bladder capacity, persistent incontinence, short penile length (J Urol 1997;157:999). Increased risk (400-fold) of adenocarcinoma of the bladder in pts with bladder exstrophy (J Urol 1970;104:699). In bladder exstrophy pts who become pregnant there is increased risk of cervical and uterine prolapse (J Urol 1978;119:478). Genital anomalies and number of surgical procedures performed may affect quality of life and interactions with others (J Urol 1999;162:2125). Rx with Latex precautions, given the number of surgical procedures they typically have

Xray: KUB demonstrates widened symphysis pubis secondary to outward rotation of innominate bones. Prenatal US: 5 factors associated with bladder exstrophy: (1) bladder never visualized, (2) lower abdominal bulge representing exstrophied bladder, (3) small penis with anteriorly placed scrotum, (4) low-set umbilical insertion, and (5) abnormal widening of iliac crests (Obstet Gynecol 1995;85:961)

Rx: Stabilization of infant. Umbilical cord should be tied close to abdominal wall to avoid irritation of the bladder mucosa. Cover exposed bladder mucosa with nonadherent film of wrap to prevent mucosa from sticking to diapers. Irrigate mucosa to keep it moist. Parental reassurance. Transfer to tertiary care center. Objectives of surgical repair: (1) abdominal wall closure, (2) urinary continence, (3) preservation of renal function, (4) reconstruction of functional and cosmetically acceptable penis in the male and external genitalia in female. Surgical repair may be achieved in a staged repair in which bladder and anterior abdominal wall are closed. Inguinal hernias usually treated at this time (BJU 1994;73:308). Some perform epispadias repair at time of bladder closure (J Urol 1996;155:300). Epispadias (if not already treated), continence-promoting procedures, and ureteral reimplantation are performed at separate intervals. Umbilical reconstruction may also be performed (J Urol 1994;151:453)

DISEASES OF THE BLADDER IN CHILDREN

9.2 CLOACAL MALFORMATIONS

Cause: Congenital anomaly; most severe form of imperforate anus with confluence of rectum, vagina, and bladder in a urogenital sinus (J Urol 1998;228:331)

Epidem: Wide spectrum of malformations; occurs in 1 in 50,00 births (J Urol 1988;228:331), persistent cloaca occurs in females only; cloacal exstrophy in 1 in 250,000 births

Pathophys: Assoc GU anomalies: vaginal duplication, vaginal agenesis, VUR

Si: Abnl-appearing perineum varying from single orifice obscured by clitoris and labia to nearly nl-appearing perineum; confluence of GI, GU, and GYN tracts may be high or low; abdominal distention; genitalia may appear ambiguous

Xray: KUB: Large fluid-filled structure in lower abdomen, often distended vagina(s) filled with urine; U/S to assess upper tracts. Sinogram to identify anatomy of urogenital sinus and relationship to bladder neck, vagina, and rectal fistula. MRI L-S spine to r/o tethered cord

Rx: Decompressive colostomy, if vagina distended and causing BOO, start CIC; rarely if CIC not successful then vesicostomy or tube vaginostomy. Endoscopic evaluation; definitive repair 6–24 mo of age (J Urol 1998;228:331)

9.3 PRUNE BELLY SYNDROME
(Eagle–Barrett Syndrome)

Cause: Most plausible etiology is that the primary defect involves intermediate and lateral mesoderm during fetal development (J Urol 1994;152:2328). Other proposed etiologies: primary urinary tract anomaly that causes bladder and ureteral dilation, which results in abdominal wall laxity; urethral obstruction early in development, which leads to urinary tract dilation and abdominal wall anomalies and recanalizes prior to birth (Peds 1984;73:470); abnl of yolk sac

Epidem: Males > females. Incidence is 1 per 35,000–50,000 live births (Am J Hum Genet 1981;33;470). May be detected as early as 15 wk gestation

Pathophys: Triad of deficiency of abdominal wall musculature, bilateral UDTs which are usually intra-abdominal, and abnl of urinary tract including dilated ureters, bladder enlargement, dilated prostatic urethra, and renal dysmorphism. Assoc abnl incl megalourethra, orthopedic, GI, respiratory, and CV abnl (J Urol 1985;133:607; J Natl Med Assoc 1973;65;327)

Sx: Usually asx unless child develops UTI

Si: Abdominal wall laxity and UDTs, often nonpalpable

Crs: Early death in those with severe pulmonary hypoplasia. 30% of survivors will develop renal failure during childhood and adolescence (J Urol 1991;145:1017; J Urol 1987;137:86)

Cmplc: Infertility. As of 1998, no reports of a male with prune belly syndrome who has sperm in his urine or semen (J Urol 1998;159:1680)

DiffDx: Posterior urethral valves, urethral atresia, high-grade VUR

Lab: Serum electrolytes, BUN, creatinine levels should be followed closely after birth

Xray: Renal US to assess degree of pelvicaliectasis, renal parenchyma, and ureteral dilation. Typical VCUG findings include enlarged smooth-walled bladder, high-grade VUR, wide open bladder neck, dilated posterior urethra

Rx: At birth, institute prophylactic abx, follow renal function closely, and obtain a renal US. Hold off instrumentation early in life due to risk of infection. VCUG should be obtained later in life. Orchidopexy also indicated. Abdominal wall plasty improves appearance, decreases psychological effects, and may improve bladder and pulmonary function (J Urol 1998;159:1675). Reimplantation indicated if child develops recurrent UTI

9.4 MYELODYSPLASIA

Cause: Unknown. Folate deficiency a risk factor (BMJ 1981;282:1509)

Epidem: 1 in 1000 births in U.S. (Peds 1982;69:511), incidence decreasing. If present in one family member, 2–5% risk of sibling being affected (Rehab Lit 1981;42:143). Most occur at lumbar vertebrae, followed by sacral, majority extend posteriorly. 85% have an Arnold–Chiari malformation: cerebellar tonsils herniating through foramen magnum, obstructing 4th ventricle

Pathophys:

Meningocele: Meninges extend beyond confines of vertebral canal

Myelomeningocele (90% lesions): Meninges, neural tissue, either nerve roots or portions of spinal cord extend beyond the vertebral canal

Lipomyelomeningocele: Protrusion of fatty tissue in addition to meninges and neural tissue

Crs: Neurologic lesion is dynamic disease process; changes may occur throughout childhood especially in infancy and during growth spurts (Jama 1987;258:1630)

Cmplc: Changes in neurologic, orthopedic, or urologic function may be sign of tethered spinal cord, syrinx, or hydromelia of the cord, increased intracranial pressure due to shunt malfunction, or partial herniation of brainstem and cerebellum. MRI best test to assess for tethered cord (Pediatr Radiol 1990;20:262). Myelodysplasia has GI, GU, orthopedic, and neurologic effects

Sx: Height of bony vertebral level and highest extent of neurologic lesion may vary from 1–3 vertebrae in one direction or another (Urology 1977;10:354)

Si: Lesion typically noted posteriorly at birth

Lab: UA, c + s, creatinine

Xray: Renal US rules out hydronephrosis and assess PVR. VCUG to r/o VUR

Urodynamics: Evaluate voiding and storage function

Rx: Closure of spine defect, then radiographic evaluation. If PVR >10–15 mL, start CIC. Urodynamics performed: Synergic—coordinated sphincter relaxation during bladder contraction or when capacity reached at end of filling; dyssynergic with or without detrusor hypertonicity—failure of relaxation or increased activity of external sphincter during bladder contraction or sustained increase in bladder pressure as bladder filled to capacity; complete denervation—no sphincteric activity noted during micturition cycle. Pts with dyssnergy at increased risk for upper tract damage are placed on CIC ± anticholinergics. Use of CIC ± anticholinergics in such patients with bladder filling pressures >40 cm H_2O and voiding pressures of >80–100 cm H_2O has decreased incidence of upper tract deterioration from 71% to 8–10% (J Urol 1995;154:1500; Am J Dis Child 1992;146:840; J Urol 1988;139:85). Periodic radiographic and urodynamic evaluation continued throughout life. Children with VUR treated same as other children with VUR. Continence may be an issue and may require augmentation to increase bladder capacity and decrease bladder pressures and/or outlet resistance procedures. Bowel regimens often necessary for fecal continence and in select cases, the Malone antegrade continence enema may be helpful (J Urol 1996;155:1416)

9.5 SACRAL AGENESIS

Cause: Uncertain; teratogenic factors may play a role

Epidem: Absence of all or part of 2 or more lower vertebral bodies, 16% affected children have mother with IDDM; 1% of IDDM mothers have a child with sacral agenesis (Urology 1983;23:506; Pediatrics 1966;37:672)

Pathophys: Affected vertebrae does not necessarily correlate with type of motor neuron lesion present

Sx: May have voiding dysfunction

Si: High arched feet, claw or hammer toes, flattened buttocks, gluteal cleft anomaly

Xray: Lateral film of spine to assess bony defect; MRI of spine: Sharp cut-off of conus

Urodynamics: 35% upper motor neuron lesion—DH, DSD (Urology 1983;23:506; J Urol 1977;118:87; Urology 1976;8:521); 40% lower motor lesion—detrusor areflexia and complete or partial denervation of external sphincter, 25% with no signs of denervation (J Urol 1994;151:1038; Urology 1983;23:506)

Crs: Injury is stable, no signs of progressive denervation

Rx: Rx based on urodynamics, aimed at preservation of upper tract

9.6 NOCTURNAL ENURESIS

Cause: No single entity explains enuresis in every child. Potential etiologies incl genetic basis, small functional bladder capacity, heavy sleeping pattern, deficiency of ADH, developmental delay, stress, psychological factors. Recent reports suggest that prostaglandins play a role in enuresis (Urology 1998;52:878)

Epidem: Affects 5–8% of children 7 yr of age, with a resolution rate of 15%/yr. If one parent was enuretic, 40% of offspring will be enuretic; if both parents were enuretic, 70% of offspring will be enuretic. 99% of children are dry by age 15 (Arch Dis Child 1974;49:259)

Pathophys: In the development of bladder and bowel control, the development of bladder control at night is the last to occur. Approximately 25% of children who attain initial nighttime control by age 12 will have a relapse and wet for a period of about 2.5 yr (Campbell's Urology 1998;7(2):2055–2068)

Sx: Asx

Si: Urinary incontinence during sleep

Crs: Spontaneous resolution common and proceeds at a rate of 15%/yr. Rx undertaken if enuresis is bothersome to child and parents

Cmplc: May adversely affect child's quality of life and lead to unnecessary punishment

DiffDx: Nocturnal enuresis without daytime component is unlikely to be related to other urologic diseases. If daytime incontinence coexists, must r/o valves in male pts, and voiding dysfunction, neurogenic bladder, and ectopic ureter in male and female pts

Lab: UA, c + s to r/o UTI, polyuria

Xray: Not indicated in primary nocturnal enuresis if the pt has a normal physical examination

Rx: Rx is initiated at age >7 yr. At this age, child, his or her peers, and parents expect dryness and wetting interferes with social activities (Scand J Urol Nephrol 1994;163(suppl):55). Restriction of evening fluids and avoiding late afternoon caffeinated products encouraged. Child should be reminded to void just before going to bed

Medical Therapy: Desmopressin acetate (DDAVP), a synthetic analog of vasopressin, stimulates kidneys to produce less urine. May be administered orally or nasally. Effect lasts 7–12 h. Dose ranges from 20–40 μg for nasal spray and 200–400 μg for oral tablet. Response may be dose dependent. DDAVP appears to be most effective at decreasing number of wet nights per wk. Its ability to produce consistent dry nights varies from 10–86% (Arch Dis Child 1987;62:674). High incidence of recurrent bedwetting upon d/c of DDAVP. Side effects of DDAVP include nasal irritation with nasal spray and less commonly water intoxication and hyponatremic seizures (Clin Pediatr 1993;special no. 19–24). When child is using DDAVP, his or her liquid intake should be restricted for the 12 h that DDAVP is functioning

Imipramine is a tricyclic antidepressant that has been demonstrated to "cure" enuresis in 50% of children and improve 80%. Relapse rate is 60% when d/c med. May exert beneficial effect by increasing bladder capacity (Ann Paeditr Fenn 1965;11:53). Generally prescribed at a dose of 25 mg for children 5–8 yr of age and 50 mg for older children. Dosage based on weight is 0.9 to 1.5 mg/kg/d (Practitioner 1971;207:809). It is typically administered shortly before child goes to bed, but may be given in late afternoon to children who wet soon after going to sleep (Can Med Assoc J 1970;102:1179). Children should take initial dose for 2 wk and adjust as needed. Infrequent side effects include personality change, adverse effects on sleep and appetite, GI sx, nervousness (Can Med Assoc J 1968;99:263; Arch Dis Child 1968;43:665). Overdosage characterized by myocardial depression and EKG changes.

Indomethacin, a cyclo-oxygenase inhibitor, is being investigated in treatment of enuresis (Urology 1998;52:878)

Behavior Modification: Should be considered as first line of rx. Responsibility reinforcements include rewarding child for dry nights and are geared to having child take an active role in the therapy. Conditioning therapy using bedwetting alarm is most effective means of treating bedwetting (Behav Res Ther 1993;31:613). Bedwetting alarm is a small battery-operated device that includes an alarm/buzzer connected to a sensory pad. Alarm is placed in the child's underwear. When pad becomes wet, the alarm/buzzer is activated. Success of this device depends on the child awakening to the alarm and getting up to complete voiding. Most important cause of failure is lack of parental understanding of typical sequence of events. Parents must be counseled that initially they will need to wake the child immediately after the alarm/buzzer goes off and have the child try to void. As time passes, the child will wake up on his or her own. Ultimately, the child will wake up prior to voiding in the bed. Time to success varies. Success rates are better than DDAVP and imipramine and are 60–80% (Campbell's Urology 1998;7(2):2055–2068)

Combination Therapy: In pts with enuresis refractory to single-modality treatment regimens, combination rx, such as bedwetting alarm plus medical rx or combined medical rx, may be used and is often successful (Eur J Pediatr 1989;148:465)

9.7 VOIDING DYSFUNCTION

Cause: Variety of etiologies (Table 9–1)
Epidem: May affect males and females. Females > males in some cases (Table 9–1)
Pathophys: See Table 9–1
Sx: See Table 9–1
Si: See Table 9–1
Lab: See Table 9–1
Xray: See Table 9–1
Other Studies: See Table 9–1
Rx: See Table 9–1

Table 9–1. Voiding Dysfunction

Type	Cause	Si/Sx	Lab/Xray	UDS	Treatment
Small-capacity hypertonic bladder	Secondary to bladder wall inflammation from recurrent UTI, may cause sensory frequency and detrusor instability	Frequency, urgency, urge incontinence, staccato voiding, nocturnal enuresis, or enuresis and dysuria	Hx (+) urine cultures; VCUG & renal US: Normal upper tracts, thick-walled bladder, small functional bladder capacity & trabeculated bladder, dilated posturethra spinning top, secondary inability to relax external sphincter	Small bladder capacity, ↑ detrusor pressure during filling, uncontrollable urge to void at capacity which sometimes can't suppress, emptying may not be complete, external sphincter may only partially relax during voiding	Elim UTI, timed voiding/double void, prophylactic abx if frequent UTI, anticholinergics if significant detrusor instability or ↓ capacity
Nonneurogenic or neurogenic bladder, Hinman–Allen syndrome (J Urol 1986;136:769)	Learned disorder, active contraction of external sphincter during voiding	Urgency urge or stress incontinence, infrequent voluntary voiding, straining to void, recurrent UTI, irregular BM with encopresis, often altered family dynamics	Hydroureteronephrosis, scarring may occur if prior UTI, 50% have severe reflux; trabeculated, large capacity bladder, ↑ PVR, constipation	Large-capacity bladder with ↓ compliance, uninhibited contraction ↑ PVR, with high-pressure voiding or ineffective detrusor contraction, intermittent flow rate, secondary inability to relax external sphincter	Timed voiding/double void, biofeedback, CIC if ↑ PVR, psychotherapy, may develop renal insufficiency if severe (Peds 1974;54:142)

Table 9-1. (cont'd)

Type	Cause	Si/Sx	Lab/Xray	UDS	Treatment
Infrequent voider "lazy bladder"	Primarily females, child learns to withhold urination for prolonged periods	May void only 1-2 x/d (Arch Dis Child 1962;37:117); normal voiding patterns as infants, occurs after toilet training, may have overflow stress incontinence, dysuria, frequency, urgency if infected	Renal bladder US, large-bladder capacity, ↑ PVR; VCUG large bladder capacity ↑ PVR, smooth walled bladder without reflux	Large capacity compliant bladder, straining to void may occur, normal EMG, intermittent stream or overflow secondary straining	Timed voiding/ double voiding, rarely CIC used; abx for UTI
Detrusor hyperreflexia	May be secondary to UTI, delayed maturation of reticulospinal pathways and inhib centers in midbrain & cerebral cortex; result of mild perinatal cerebral insult; rarely associated with significant constipation (Clin Nephrol 1985;5:154)	Frequency, urgency, urge incontinence, Vincent's curtsy	Xray, mildly trabec, or thick-walled bladder	Uninhibited bladder contractions during filling, which child may not sense or abolish by ↑ activity of external sphincter (Urol Clin North Am 1980;7:321; Neurourol Urodynam 1991;10:169)	Anticholinergics, treat infections if present

10 Diseases of the Urethra in Children

10.1 POSTERIOR URETHRAL VALVES

Cause: Congenital anomaly that leads to urinary outflow obstruction. Three types of valves have been described. Type I: A pair of leaflets that pass downward and laterally from lower border of verumontanum and extend around membranous urethra to fuse anteriorly at the 12:00 position. Type II: Folds that arise from verumontanum and proceed proximally to divide into membranes; these are thought to be nonobstructive. Type III: Centrally perforated diaphragms not related to verumontanum and may be cephalad or caudad to verumontanum (J Urol 1919;3:289)

Epidem: Most common cause of urinary outflow obstruction in pediatric population (J Pediatr Surg 1983;18:70). Incidence estimated at 1 in 5000–8000 male births. Accounts for about 10% of cases of prenatally diagnosed hydronephrosis (Am J Roentgenol 1987;148:1959)

Pathophys: Most plausible etiology of type I urethral valves is a failure of regression of venterolateral folds of urogenital sinus during fetal development. Type I valves may be partially disrupted type II valves (Pediatr Surg Int 1992;8:45). Type III valves are probably the result of persistence of urogenital membrane during development. Congenital urethral obstruction occurs early in second trimester, after remainder of urinary tract has differentiated. Maturation of urinary tract occurs in the setting of elevated bladder and urethral pressures, which may alter development of upper urinary tract. With severe obstruction, there may be oligohydramnios and pulmonary hypoplasia.

Assoc GU abnl incl VUR in 50% of cases (J Urol 1982;128:994; BJU 1979;51:100) and UDT in 12% (J Urol 1980;124:101)

Sx: If oligohydramnios was present the infant may develop respiratory distress

Si: Prenatal US demonstrating bilateral hydronephrosis in the male infant, confirmed postnatal, delayed voiding longer than 24 h after birth, palpable distended bladder, excessive thirst, polyuria, failure to thrive, dehydration. Older children may present with hematuria, incontinence, and recurrent UTI. Pneumothorax on chest Xray in newborn with respiratory problems

Crs: Prenatal US has allowed for earlier detection of posterior urethral valves, but has not improved clinical outcome (J Urol 1992;148:125). In utero rx for posterior urethral valves and its consequences are still considered investigational and should be performed at select institutions. Children with posterior urethral valves diagnosed at birth are at higher risk for renal failure than those who have the condition diagnosed later in life. Good prognostic factors include serum creatinine (<0.8 ng/dL after age 1 yr), VURD syndrome, urinary ascites, and a large bladder (J Urol 1990;144:1209; J Urol 1988;140:993). Of surviving infants with posterior urethral valves, 25–40% will develop end-stage renal disease (J Urol 1994;151:275; BJU 1985;57:7). Of those who develop end-stage renal disease, 1/3 will do so soon after birth and the remainder in their teenage years (Smith GHH, Duckett JW. Urethral lesions in infants and children. In Adult and Pediatric Urology, 3rd ed. St. Louis: Mosby Yearbook, 1996: 2411). Renal transplantation is an option for these children, but cmplc of renal transplantation higher in children under age 2 (J Pediatr Surg 1992;27:629; J Urol 1988;140:1129)

Cmplc: Growth failure related to renal insufficiency and possible impaired sexual function and reduced fertility related to renal insufficiency and surgical rx

DiffDx: Bilateral hydronephrosis on pre- and postnatal US carries diffdx of prune belly syndrome, urethral atresia, high-grade VUR, bilateral UPJO, and bilateral UVJ obstruction

Lab: Serum electrolytes, BUN, creatinine levels. Immediately after birth the infant's serum creatinine level will reflect the mother's creatinine and typically equilibrates in the next 96 h (Urol Clin North Am 1990;17:343). UA, c + s, infants with respiratory distress need ABG

Xray: Renal/bladder US is obtained to look for posterior urethral dilation, bladder size, wall thickness, ureteral dilation, and hydronephrosis, and to assess renal parenchymal echogenicity and thickness and corticomedullary junction. Increased renal echogenicity on US suggests renal dysfunction (Radiology 1988;167:623). Lack of distinction of corticomedullary junction also suggests altered renal function (J Urol 1992;148:122). VCUG is gold standard for diagnosing posterior urethral valves. Typical findings include dilated posterior urethra with U-shaped cutoff at level of membranous urethra, often with incomplete bladder emptying (Gillenwater JY, Grayhack, T Howards SS, et al, eds. Adult and Pediatric Urology, 3rd ed. St. Louis: Mosby Yearbook, 1996). Additional radiologic imaging such as renal scans may be indicated to assess renal function

Rx: Initial rx involves stabilizing infant with correction of acidosis, underlying electrolyte abnormalities, infection, and respiratory issues if present. Immediate drainage via an 8-Fr feeding tube should be performed. Catheter placement may be difficult due to coiling of tube in dilated posterior urethra and bladder neck hypertrophy. Once infant is stabilized and serum creatinine followed, proceed with endoscopic valve ablation. Early valve ablation within first months of life may result in recovery of normal bladder function and appearance (J Urol 1997;157:984)

If infant's urethra is too small to pass an 8-Fr cystoscope, temporary cutaneous vesicostomy may be performed (J Urol 1990;144:1212; Urol Clin North Am 1974;1:484). Should see improvement in serum creatinine after primary valve ablation. If creatinine does not improve after valve ablation, vesicostomy or use of high diversion indicated. Use of high diversion is controversial (J Urol 1997;158:1008; Urol Clin North Am 1980;7:265)

Subsequent urodynamic evaluation is helpful in assessing bladder function in valve pts and in planning rx regimens (J Urol 1997;158:1011). Urodynamic abnl present in 20–88% of pts after valve ablation (J Urol 1990;144:122; Urol Clin North Am 1990;17:3737; J Urol 1979;121:769). Such findings include myogenic failure, DI, and decreased bladder compliance. Children with myogenic failure are initially rx with timed voiding and double or triple void regimens, while those with DI and decreased compliance may benefit from anticholinergic therapy. Pts with significant myogenic failure may require CIC to empty their bladders. Pts with refractory poor compliance may require bladder augmentation

Children with VUR should be started on prophylactic abx. Coexistent VUR will resolve in 20% of cases after valve ablation (J Urol 1990;144:1209). Ureteral reimplantation indicated for children with breakthrough infections, but this carries a 15–30% cmplc rate (J Urol 1985;133:240; AUA Update Series 1983;2:1). VURD (valve unilateral reflux and dysplasia syndrome) is seen with unilateral high-grade VUR in valve pts. Such children often have better renal function as a result of the "pop-off" effect of the VUR, and will ultimately require ipsilateral nephroureterectomy, the timing of which is controversial. The dilated ureter may be used to augment bladder if augmentation is indicated (J Urol 1997;158:1011)

10.2 ANTERIOR URETHRAL VALVES

Cause: Congenital anomaly

Epidem: Rare lesion. Present earlier if obstruction is severe. May be detected prenatally

Pathophys: May be secondary to aborted attempt at urethral duplication, failure of alignment of distal and proximal urethra, or cystic dilation of periurethral glands (J Urol 1987;138:1211; BJU 1969;41:228)

Sx: Urinary retention, urethrorrhagia

Si: Pelvicaliectasis, VUR, poor urinary stream, failure to thrive

Crs: Better prognosis than posterior urethral valves. Chronic renal insufficiency in <5% patients (J Urol 1997;158:1030)

Lab: Serum electrolytes, BUN, creatinine, urine c + s to r/o UTI

Xray: Renal US to assess pelvicaliectasis; VCUG: Urethra dilated proximal to valve and narrow distal to it

Rx: Varies with timing of presentation, severity of obstruction and diverticular versus phallic size. Initial rx, urinary tract decompression with catheter. If urethra size is adequate, valve fulguration or one-stage urethroplasty. If there is a large urethral diverticulum, staged urethroplasty. In the setting of high-grade VUR or persistent azotemia consider vesicostomy as initial rx (J Urol 1997;158:1030)

10.3 HYPOSPADIAS

Cause: Embryologic maldevelopment. May be related to failure of urethral folds to coalesce in the midline in more proximal forms of hypospadias, and lack of canalization of glans channel in distal forms of hypospadias

Epidem: Incidence is 1 in 300 live male births (Mayo Clin Proc 1974;49:52). Distal (anterior) hypospadias occurs in approximately 50% of affected males, middle in 30% of affected males, and proximal (posterior) in 20% of affected males (Fig. 10–1) (J Urol 1992;147:665)

Assoc Anomalies: Chordee (penile curvature), UDT in 9% of affected males (Urol Clin North Am 1981;8:565). In perineal and penoscrotal hypospadias there is a 10–15% incidence of prostatic utricles (J Urol 1980;123:407). Intersex abnl assoc with hypospadias incl adrenogenital syndrome, mixed gonadal dysgenesis, Reifenstein syndrome, 5-alpha-reductase deficiency, true hermaphrodite, and micropenis

Sx: Asx

Si: Urethral meatal opening proximal to tip of the penis. Typically, ventral prepuce is deficient but may be present in the setting of megameatus intact prepuce variant of hypospadias. Penile curvature (chordee) may be present. Meatus may appear stenotic

Crs: If left untreated, may affect ability to void with a straight stream and to have forward-directed flow of semen. Chordee, if severe and not treated, may prevent intercourse

Cmplc: Incidence of surgical cmplc varies with location of hypospadiac meatus and incl wound dehiscence and infection, meatal regression, urethrocutaneous fistula, urethral diverticulum, residual chordee, urethral stricture, meatal stenosis, BXO, excess penile shaft skin (Urol Clin North Am 1980;7:443)

Lab: If testes not palpable, r/o intersex anomaly

Xrays: Not indicated unless other congenital anomalies suspected

Rx: Surgery indicated to bring urethral meatus to tip of penis, treat chordee if present, create conical-appearing glans, and correct scrotal abnormality if present. Also, removal of asymmetric prepuce allows for more nl-appearing phallus. Type of surgery performed varies with meatal location and surgeon's preference. Distal and middle forms of hypospadias more commonly repaired

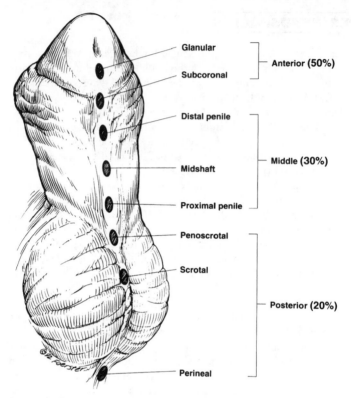

Figure 10–1. Locations of hypospadiac meatus. (Reproduced from Duckett JW. Successful hypospadias repair. Contemporary Urology 1992;4:42–55. Copyright by Medical Economics.)

using Snodgrass modification of Thiersch–Duplay repair (J Urol 1994;151: 464). More proximal forms may be similarly treated or via use of transverse island flaps (J Urol 1998;159:2129; Urol Clin North Am 1980;7:423). Surgery usually performed at around 6 mo to 1 yr of age to minimize effect of separation anxiety between infant and parents, and to not interfere with toilet training

10.4 EPISPADIAS

Cause: Congenital anomaly identified at birth

Epidemic: Male:female 3–4:1 (Urol Clin North Am 1978;5:107). Isolated male epispadias incidence of 1 in 118,000 live male births (J Urol 1949;52:513). 90% cases assoc with bladder exstrophy, which occurs 1 in 50,000 live births (Urol Clin North Am 1978;5:107). Female epispadias rare (1 in 480,000 female births) (J Urol 1949;62:513)

Pathophys: In males, most common is penopubic. Defect begins at bladder neck and involves length of phallus and urethral plate. Assoc with urinary incontinence. Dorsal chordee (curvature) secondary to intrinsic deformity of corporeal bodies (J Urol 1984;132:1122). More distal forms (penile and balanitic) assoc with less urinary incontinence. Female epispadias may vary from patulous urethra involving bladder neck to dorsally split and cleft urethra

Sx: Asx

Si: Dorsally located urethral meatus, chordee

Cmplc: Urinary incontinence

DiffDx: Bladder exstrophy/epispadias complex

Rx: Surgical repair. Goal is straight penis with ventrally located urethral meatus and phallic skin coverage in cosmetically appealing manner. Majority of males with penopubic epispadias and some with penile epispadias require bladder neck reconstruction for urinary incontinence. Rarely, bladder augmentation indicated for small bladder capacity and persistent incontinence

10.5 URETHRAL POLYP

Cause: Benign neoplasm

Epidem: Rare lesion in male children, prostatic urethra most common, rarely seen in anterior urethra (Urology 1991;38:143)

Pathophys: ? Secondary to developmental error in invagination process of submucous glanular material of inner zone of prostate (BJU 1993;72:937)

Sx: Strangury, obstructive voiding symptoms

Si: Hematuria
DiffDx: Sarcoma botryoides, prominent verumontanum of prostate
Lab: Urine for UA, c + s
Xray: VCUG confirms dx
Rx: Transurethral excision (Urology 1994;44:106)

10.6 URETHRAL PROLAPSE

Cause: Urethral prolapse is a circular eversion of the mucosa at urethral meatus. Exact cause not known. Possible etiologies incl excessive urethral mobility, significant mucosal redundancy, increased abdominal pressure, infection, neuromuscular deficiency, or poor attachments between muscular layers of the urethra (J Urol 1986;135:100)

Epidem: Black girls > white girls (J Urol 1986;135:100). Incidence estimated at 1 in 3000 (J Urol 1987;137:115). Peak age of occurrence is 5–8 yr

Pathophys: Prolapse of urethral mucosa leads to congestion and edema. Often present with genital bleeding, may progress to necrosis of affected mucosa

Sx: Dysuria and discomfort

Si: Doughnut-shaped anterior vulvar mass that completely encircles urethral meatus. If in question, gentle probing of urethral meatus with pediatric feeding tube will demonstrate circular nature, bleeding, and urinary retention

Crs: May progress to necrosis of affected urethral mucosa

Cmplc: Necrosis of mucosa

DiffDx: Prolapsed ureterocele, periurethral cyst, Gartner's duct cyst, sarcoma botryoides, prolapsed urethral polyp, ectopic ureter, hydrometrocolpos, condyloma accuminata, periurethral abscess, bladder prolapse (J Peds 1998;133:552)

Lab: UA, c + s

Xray: Not indicated unless another disease process is suspected

Rx: Conservative rx may be attempted initially with oral abx, estrogen cream, and sitz baths (BJU 1993;72:503; Obstet Gynecol 1982;59:69). Complete resolution may take 1–4 wk. If conservative rx fails or there is tissue necrosis, cystoscopy and excision of redundant urethral mucosa indicated

10.7 MEATAL STENOSIS

Cause: Thought to be related to a nonspecific inflammation of urethral meatus (Postgrad Med 1992;91:237) or ischemia of meatal mucosa

Epidem: May be most common cmplc of circumcision (Postgrad Med 1992;91:237). True incidence is unclear. Occurs in circumcised males. Onset of sx after circumcision varies from 4 mo to 13 yrs (BJU 1995;75:91; NZ Med J 1998;111: 57–58)

Sx: Acute penile or glanular pain at start of voiding

Si: Narrow, high-velocity urinary stream, urinary frequency, pinhole urethral meatus with lower margins bridged by thin filmy membrane (BJU 1995;75:91), hematuria

Lab: Urine c + s to r/o UTI

Rx: Meatotomy may be done in office using topical anesthesia (EMLA) or under anesthesia

11 Diseases of the Penis in Children

11.1 PHIMOSIS

Cause: At birth a physiologic phimosis is present in the majority of infants due to preputial adhesions

Epidem: By age 3 yr, 90% of foreskins are retractable; <1% of males have phimosis by age 17 (Arch Dis Child 1968;43:200)

Pathophys: Phimosis in infants is physiologic. During the first few yr, as penis grows, accumulation of epithelial debris (smegma) occurs under prepuce which separates preputial adhesions. Rarely, a cicatricial preputial ring may form, preventing spontaneous retraction

Sx: Usually asx. If irritation present, may develop pain, bleeding, dysuria

Si: Ballooning of foreskin with voiding, inability to retract foreskin fully, smegma pearls, balanitis, and balanoposthitis can occur

Crs: Often resolves by 3–5 yr of age

Cmplc: Increased incidence of penile cancer in uncircumcised males with poor personal hygiene. Increased risk of STDs

Lab: UA, c + s if UTI suspected

Xray: Not routinely indicated

Rx: Rx of congenital phimosis not routinely indicated until age 4–5 yr, at which time spontaneous retraction should occur. Indications for circumcision include history of UTI and VUR, recurrent UTI, persistent phimosis, recurrent balanitis and balanoposthitis, and parental desire (parents should be counseled about indications and risks of circumcision). Cmplc rate for neonatal circumcision is 0.2–3% (Ross JH. Circumcision: Pro and con. In: Elder JS, ed. Pediatric Urology for the General Urologist. New York: Igaku-

Shoin, 1996:49). Contraindications to neonatal circumcision include coexisting hypospadias, chordee without hypospadias, webbed penis, small penis, and dorsal hood deformity. Infants with a large hernia or hydrocele are more likely to develop buried penis and secondary phimosis if circumcision is performed prior to rx of hernia/hydrocele (Campbell's Urology 1998;7(2):2120–2143). Topical steroid cream (0.05% betamethasone cream) has up to a 95% success rate in small series (BJU 1996;78:786; J Urol 1999;162:1162)

11.2 PARAPHIMOSIS

Cause: Prolonged retraction of foreskin
Epidem: Occurs in uncircumcised males
Sx: Penile pain
Si: Penile swelling, phimotic ring
Cmplc: Infection, ischemia, tends to recur
Rx: Reduce: Gentle, steady pressure to foreskin to reduce swelling and then pull foreskin back over glans (BMJ 1996;312:838). If prolonged, then dorsal slit or circumcision may be indicated

11.3 MICROPENIS

Cause: Deficiency of gonadotropic hormones occuring after 14 wk gestation. Most common causes include hypogonadotropic hypogonadism (Kallmann's syndrome, Prader–Willi syndrome, Laurence–Moon–Biedl syndrome), hypergonadotropic hypogonadism (primary testicular failure), and idiopathic factors (Johns Hopkins Med J 1980;146:156). Failure of hypothalamus to produce adequate amount of GnRH is most common cause. May be seen in association with chromosomal abnls such as Klinefelter's syndrome (47XXY), other poly-X syndromes, and abnls involving chromosomes 8,13, and 18 (J Urol 1994;152:4)
Pathophys: Defined as a normally formed penis at least 2.5 standard deviations below the mean in size. Penis of a newborn should be at least 1.9 cm long (J Urol 1994;152:4)

Sx: Asx

Si: Stretched penile length is <2.0 cm in the newborn or at least 2 standard deviations below the mean in older child. May be assoc with small scrotum, small testes, or UDTs

Crs: Identified most commonly in infancy. Ultimate penile size may not be nl but majority of pts will have adequate length for penile function

Cmplc: Inadequate adult penile length. Use of extensive androgen rx before puberty may reduce eventual penile size (J Urol 1994;152)

DiffDx: Small but nl-length phallus, intersex if UDTs

Lab: Karyotype should be performed on all pts. Testosterone levels should be taken before and after HCG stimulation. If pituitary abnl suspected, perform serial serum glucose, Na^+, K^+, serum cortisol, thyroid function tests

Xray: MRI to assess hypothalamus, pituitary, midline brain structures

Rx: Androgen therapy to assess penile response: testosterone enanthate 25 mg im every mo for 3 mo or transdermal testosterone. Poor prognosis if penile length does not increase in response to hormone therapy (J Urol 1993;150:657). Some advocate gender reassignment if no response to androgen therapy (Campbells' Urology 1998;7(69):2120–2143), very controversial at present

12 Diseases of the Testes and Scrotum in Children

12.1 CRYPTORCHIDISM (UNDESCENDED TESTICLE)

Cause: Abnl of testicular descent

Epidem: One of most common disorders of childhood; affects 3.4% of full-term infants and 30% of premature infants (Scorer CG, Farrington GH. Congenital Deformities of the Testis and Epididymis. New York: Appleton-Century Crofts, 1971). At age 1 yr, incidence is 0.8–1.5% (Pediatrics 1993;92:44). In 10% of children, defect is bilateral (Scorer & Farrington, 1971). 3.5% of cryptorchid testes will be absent (J Urol 1974;111:840)

Pathophys: Proposed etiologies of testicular descent incl (1) traction of testis by gubernaculum and/or cremasteric muscle, (2) differential growth of body wall in relation to gubernaculum, (3) intra-abdominal pressure pushing testis through inguinal canal, (4) effect of genitofemoral nerve. These may play a role in testicular descent, but endocrine factors appear to play the major role (Endocrinology 1991;129:741, 1409)

Sx: Asx

Si: Empty hemiscrotum, testis palpable or nonpalpable in inguinal canal or other sites of ectopia. Size of ipsilateral scrotum may be diminished

Crs: If undescended testicle (UDT) is going to descend spontaneously, it often does so within the first yr of life, with most descending by 6 mo of age. After age 1 yr, low likelihood of spontaneous descent

Cmplc: Testicular cancer: 10% of testicular tumors arise from UDTs (BJU 1992;70:656). UDT 35–48 times more likely than nl testis to undergo malignant degeneration (J Urol 1975;114:77). UDTs have increased risk of testicular torsion. There is risk of a symptomatic hernia, as the processus vaginalis remains patent with UDT. Infertility: The higher and longer the testis resides away from the scrotum, the greater the risk of damage to seminiferous tubules (J Urol 1995;153:1255). Assoc abnl of vas deferens and epididymis may affect subsequent fertility (Urol Clin North Am 1982;9:339)

DiffDx: Vanished testis, retractile testis, intersex abnormality in children with bilateral nonpalpable testes, and crytporchidsm may be assoc with Klinefelter's syndrome, hypogonadotropic hypogonadism, prune belly syndrome, myelomeningocele, hypospadias, Wilms' tumor, Noonan's syndrome, Prader–Willi syndrome, cystic fibrosis

Lab: Not routinely indicated. Serum testosterone, LH, and FSH levels in children with bilateral nonpalpable UDTs. Other labs indicated if assoc abnl suspected

Xray: Not indicated

Rx: Aimed at bringing testis into dependent position in scrotum ideally by age 1 yr. Medical and surgical therapies may be used. Medical: HCG and GnRH. The International Health Foundation recommendations for HCG rx are biweekly injections of 250 IU for infants, 500 IU for children up to 6 yr of age, and 1000 IU for those ≥6 yr of age, for a total of 5 wk. GnRH at 1.2 mg/d as nasal spray for 4 wk successful in 6.18–70% of pts (Int J Urol 1992;15:135; Urol Clin North Am 1982;9:413; Klin Paediatr 1981;193:382; J Urol 1977;118:985). Surgical rx includes laparoscopy, a useful diagnostic and therapeutic tool in the setting of a nonpalpable testis (Am Surg 1994;60:143; J Urol 1994;152:1249). If testis is palpable, inguinal approach is used and testis placed in subdartos scrotal pouch. Surgical cmplc incl infection, injury to testicular vessels and/or vas deferens, and testicular ascent

12.2 PEDIATRIC HYDROCELE

Cause: Collection of fluid between parietal and visceral layers of the tunica albuginea

Epidem: Present in 6% of full-term boys. Risk of clinically evident contralateral hydrocele or hernia after unilateral repair is 7% (J Urol 1999;162:1169)

Pathophys: Patent processus vaginalis allows peritoneal fluid to pass into tunica vaginalis

Sx: Typically asx

Si: Scrotal swelling that transilluminates; if a communicating hydrocele (patent processus vaginalis), then the scrotal swelling may fluctuate throughout the day

Crs: May resolve spontaneously within the first yr of life

Cmplc: If processus vaginalis remains patent may develop inguinal hernia

DiffDx: Inguinal hernia, testicular torsion, and testicular tumor

Xray: If testis is not palpable due to the size of the hydrocele, scrotal US will evaluate testes and confirm presence of hydrocele

Rx: If the hydrocele remains after the child is 1 yr old, or if it is communicating hydrocele or assoc with an inguinal hernia, inguinal exploration, ligation of the patent processus vaginalis, and drainage of the hydrocele are indicated

12.3 PEDIATRIC INGUINAL HERNIA

Cause: Patent processus vaginalis allows peritoneal contents to pass into inguinal canal. May also be related to abnl collagen synthesis in inguinal area (Ann Surg 1993;218:754)

Epidem: Majority of pediatric hernias present within first yr of life. Overall incidence 1–4.4%. Premature infants have increased risk of 13%. Male > females. 6–10% of children with unilateral hernia will develop clinical hernia on contralateral side (J Pediatr Surg 1993;28:1026). Of girls presenting with inguinal hernias, 1.6% are 46XY with an intra-abdominal testes (see 13.2)

Pathophys: Incomplete closure of patent processus vaginalis during development. Hernia may contain intestine, omentum, or ovary

Crs: Risk of incarceration highest in children <1 yr (J Pediatr Surg 1993;28:582)

Sx: May be asx. Pain, N/V, abdominal distention may be present if incarceration occurs

Si: Inguinal groin bulge

Cmplc: Incarceration, ischemia to testis related to compression of testicular vessels, and injury to the testicular vessels and/or vas deferens during surgery

DiffDx: Hydrocele

Lab: Karyotype recommended for all girls presenting with an inguinal hernia

Xray: Not routinely indicated

Rx: Inguinal exploration, reduction of the hernia, ligation of processus vaginalis

12.4 YOLK SAC TUMOR

Cause: Malignant neoplasm

Epidem: Most common testis tumor in infants and children. 60% of germ cell tumors in prepubertal boys; 30% occur within first 2 yr of life (J Urol 1988;140:1109; Am J Clin Pathol 1984;81:427; Cancer 1980;46:1213). 1.04 per 1 million (Eur Urol 1984;10:73); 1.5% of adult germ cell tumors (Virchow Arch (A) 1982;396:247)

Pathophys: May arise from extraembryonic yolk sac structures (Cancer 1977;39:162; Human Pathol 1976;7:675). Histopath: Schiller–Duval body

Sx: Often painless

Si: Testicular enlargement

DiffDx: Other germ cell tumors, epidermoid tumor

Lab: Elevated serum AFP: Sensitive marker in initial dx and in f/up for mets (Urol Clin North Am 1993;20:67). Increased AFP may be seen in nl infants up to 2 yr old (Urol Clin North Am 1993;20:7). BetaHCG and CEA may be increased but not reliable enough as markers (Eur Urol 1984;10:73)

Xray: Scrotal US: Intratesticular mass; CT scan abd/pelvis to r/o retroperitoneal disease; C-xray to r/o pulmonary mets

Rx: Initial rx: Radical inguinal orchiectomy. Subsequent rx: If CT (−) and C-xray (−), AFP normalizes postorchiectomy—follow with serial AFPs and radiologic studies. 10–20% relapse rate (J Pediatr Surg 1986;21:108). If AFP remains elevated and CT (–) and (–) mets, then RPLND (Cancer Treat Rev 1983;10:265). If AFP elevated and CT with limited retroperitoneal disease, may benefit from RPLND (J Urol 1987;137:954). If bulky retroperitoneal disease or other areas of mets, chemotherapy indicated

12.5 RHABDOMYOSARCOMA

Cause: Malignant lesion arising from embryonal mesenchyme. Small round tumor

Epidem: Most common soft-tissue sarcoma in children, annual incidence 1.3–4.4/million. GU sites incl prostate, bladder, vagina, pelvic, paratesticular (NCI monograph 1981;56:61). Male:female 1.4:1; peaks at 2–6 yr and 15–19 yr (Cancer 1970;25:1384; 1997;40:2015). Increased incidence with neurofibromatosis (J Urol 1995;154:1516)

Pathophys: Embryonal most common type. Histopath: Unencapsulated and infiltrative. Staging: Pre-rx

    Stage I: All favorable sites, nonmetastatic

    Stage II: All favorable sites, primary tumor <5 cm, (–) nodes, nonmetastatic

    Stage III: All unfavorable sites, primary tumor >5 cm, and/or (–) nodes

    Stage IV: All metastatic disease

Si: Vary with site and size: Urinary retention, hematuria, foul-smelling discharge

Sx: Vary with site and size: Strangury, incontinence

Crs: Rapid growth and invasion of soft tissue: May spread via lymphatics or blood

Lab: US bladder: May show lesion; US scrotum: Paratesticular or cord lesion

Cysto/vaginoscopy: Visualization of lesion and bx

Xray: CT abd/pelvis to assess for mets, nodal disease. May be able to percutaneously bx pelvic mass under CT guidance

Rx: Paratesticular: Radical orchiectomy; (–) nodes then chemo; if (+) nodes then RPLND. XRT added to chemo if (+) nodes or microscopic residual disease (J Urol 1998;159:1031).

Pelvic/bladder/vaginal/prostate: Bx to establish dx and determine histology—bx palpable nodes. Primary therapy chemo and XRT. Exenerative surgery reserved for failures (J Urol 1995;154:5405). Limited excisional surgery if tumor involves anterior wall of bladder or dome

12.6 TESTICULAR TORSION

Cause: Neonatal torsion is an extravaginal torsion and caused by lack of fixation of the gubernaculum, which allows testis, epididymis, and tunica vaginalis to rotate within the scrotum. Pubertal torsion is an intravaginal torsion. Gubernaculum is fixed to scrotal wall and torsion occurs due to a narrow mesenteric attachment from the cord onto the testis and epididymis, the bell-clapper abnl (Urology 1994;44:144)

Epidem: May occur at any age, but most common during adolescence. Incidence about 1 in 4000 male pts under age 25 (J Urol 1989;142:746). With intravaginal torsion there is increased risk of torsion of contralateral testis (Br J Surg 1974;61:905)

Pathophys: Initial obstruction of venous drainage with secondary edema and hemorrhage and subsequent arterial obstruction

Sx: In the infant, sx may be absent or infant may present with irritability and restlessness. In the adolescent, sx include testicular pain, N/V

Si: Scrotal swelling, absent cremasteric reflexes, reactive hydrocele, abnormal testicular lie

Crs: Good prognosis if treated within 4–6 h of onset (BJU 1978;50:43). If untreated, will lead to testicular loss

Cmplc: Testicular loss and fertility may be affected in the pubertal or postpubertal male (J Urol 1980;124:375)

DiffDx: Incarcerated hernia, hematocele, hydrocele, testicular tumor, idiopathic scrotal edema, torsion of a testicular/epididymal appendage, epididymitis/orchitis

Lab: UA; if abnl, c + s

Xray: Scrotal US with Doppler study or nuclear perfusion study may help confirm clinical suspicion

Rx: Dx of testicular torsion is clinical. If cannot r/o torsion, scrotal exploration warranted. Rx is scrotal exploration. Testis removed if it remains ischemic/necrotic after detorsion, and contralateral scrotal orchidopexy performed. If affected testis appears viable after detorsion, orchidopexy is performed (J Urol 1989;142:746)

12.7 TORSION OF THE TESTICULAR APPENDAGES

Cause: Twisting of the appendix testis or appendix epididymis on its vascular supply

Epidem: Appendix testis more commonly affected than appendix epididymis (Pediatr Med Chir 1994;16:521)

Pathophys: Twisting of appendage on its vascular supply causes venous obstruction, edema, and subsequent arterial obstruction

Sx: Scrotal pain. Often, child can point to localize the pain to the area superior to the testis

Si: Scrotal swelling, reactive hydrocele, blue dot sign (Urology 1973;1:63)

Crs: If left untreated, torsed appendage will become ischemic and involute and may calcify

DiffDx: Testicular torsion, epididymitis, orchitis

Lab: UA, c + s

Xray: Scrotal US with Doppler helps identify enlarged, edematous appendage and demonstrates good blood flow to the ipsilateral testis

Rx: Supportive: If child can be made comfortable with pain medication, no exploration needed. If cannot r/o torsion, exploration and excision of the appendage indicated

13 Other Diseases in Children

13.1 NEUROBLASTOMA

Cause: Malignancy arising from cells of neural crest that form sympathetic ganglia and adrenal medulla

Epidem: Most common malignant tumor of infancy (J Pediatr 1975;86:254). 6–8% of all childhood malignancies; 50% occur in children <2 yr of age and >75% in children <4 yr (Ann Surg 1968;167:132; J Pediatr Surg 1969;4:244). Up to 70% have mets at time of dx. Bone marrow frequently involved (50%). Liver mets common in younger children and bone mets common in older children. (Am J Dis Child 1970;119:49)

Pathophys:

Histopath: One of the small round cell tumors of childhood; cells may clump and form rosettes. Located anywhere along sympathetic chain; >50% are in abdomen and 2/3 of these arise in adrenal gland. Staging:

Stage 0:   Neuroblastoma in-situ

Stage I: Tumor confined to structure or organ of origin

Stage II: Tumor extends in continuity beyond organ or structure of origin but does not cross the midline. Ispilateral regional nodes may be involved

Stage III: Tumor extends in continuity beyond the midline. Bilateral regional nodes may be involved

Stage IV: Distant mets involving bone, bone marrow, brain, skin, liver, lung, soft tissues, or distant lymph nodes

Stage IV-S: Pts who would be otherwise classified as a stage I or II disease but who have remote spread of tumor confined to one or more of following sites: liver, skin, or bone marrow (without x-ray evidence of bone mets on skeletal survey) (Cancer 1971;27:374)

Sx: Bone pain, irritability

Si: Abdominal mass, fever, generalized malaise, anorexia, weight loss, pallor, subcutaneous nodes, periorbital mets common, intractable diarrhea secondary to VIP production, acute myoclonic encephalopathy, signs of catecholamine secretion, syndrome mimicking erythroblastosis

DiffDx: Wilms' tumor

Crs: Assoc with neurofibromatosis and Hirschsprung's disease (Cancer 1966;19:1032; Am J Roentgenol 1965;95:217)

Lab: CBC: usually nl, with mets anemia and thrombocytopenia, ESR usually elevated with mets. Bone marrow aspiration: pos in up to 70% (Am J Dis Child 1970;119:49). Urinary catecholamine: 95% have increased levels of VMA, HVA, or both; 24-h urine quantification most accurate

Xray: C-xray to r/o pulmonary mets, thoracic tumor, tumor extension into posterior mediastinum; KUB may demonstrate mass with stippled calcifications. CT scan helps distinguish neuroblastoma from Wilms' tumor. Bone scan to r/o bony mets

Rx: If well-localized favorable disease, surgical removal. If unfavorable disease, bx to confirm dx then give chemotherapy, consolidation, second-look surgery, XRT and MIBG followed by high-dose chemo with or without TBI and rescue with pt's own harvested bone marrow or bone marrow from HLA-matched sibling. 2-yr survival up to 40% in those with unfavorable disease/recurrent disease with BMT (J Clin Oncol 1984;2:609). Stage IV-S: Observe; high likelihood disease will spontaneously regress

13.2 INTERSEX

Dialogues Pediatr Urol 2000;23:1

Cause: Congenital anomaly

Epidem: May be secondary to CAH, maternal steroid use or adrenal tumor, chromosomal abnl, or receptor defects. Deficiency of 21-hydroxylase responsible for 95% cases of CAH

Pathophys: Indications for evaluation: Ambiguous genitalia such that cannot tell sex at all. In female: clitoral hypertrophy, skin fused labia, palpable gonad; in male: bilateral impalpable testes, severe hypospadias, hypospadias with UDT

Si/Sx: See Table 13–1

Lab: Buccal smear detects presence of Barr body, which represents 2nd X chromosome-limited, only detects Barr bodies in 30% cells examined. FISH: Staining of lymphocytes to identify X and Y chromosomes, more rapid, less expensive than karyotyping. Karyotype-G-banded karyotyping: Minimum of 30 lymphocytes examined to exclude mosaicism with 95% probability; expensive, time consuming. Gene probe may help make definitive dx by identifying gene mutations and deletions. Biochemical evaluation: See Table 13–1

Xray: US pelvis to identify if uterus present; US of palpable gonad can help identify testis and dysgenetic testes; presence of a cyst within gonad suggests ovotestis. US abdomen to assess adrenals, r/o tumor or massive enlargement. Genitogram helpful in females with CAH to delineate level at which vagina opens into urogenital sinus

Rx: See Table 13–1

13.3 VAGINAL AGENESIS

Cause: Incomplete or absent canalization of vaginal plate

Epidem: Occurs in 1 of 4000–5000 females. Second most common cause of primary infertility in females (Clin Obstet Gynecol 1987;30:682)

Pathophys: Normal vaginal plate canalization occurs at wk 11 of gestation and is completed by wk 20. Uterus is present but often rudimentary without a lumen. 1/3 of affected females have renal abnl, most commonly renal agenesis (Mayer–Rokitansky–Küster–Hauser syndrome) or renal ectopia (Ann IM 1976;85:224). Renal fusion abnl such as horseshoe kidney may also occur. 12% will have skeletal anomalies (Ann IM 1976;85:224). Also assoc with McKusick–Kaufman hydrometrocolpos–polydactyly syndrome (Am J Dis Child 1987;141:1133)

Sx: Amenorrhea

Si: Vagina may be absent or consist of a shallow (2–3 cm) pouch

Table 13-1. Intersex Disorders

Disorder	Chromosomes	Presentation	Laboratory	Complications	Treatment
Klinefelter's syndrome	47XXY, 46XX; 47XXY, 48XXXY, 49XXXXY, 46XX (sex reversal-detectable Y DNA)	Small, firm testes <2 cm wide/diameter; poor muscle development and female body fat distribution	Serum testosterone level 1/2 nl; ↑ LH and FSH, 50–75% with XXY have gynecomastia; seminif tubule dysgenesis (J Clin Endocrinol 1942;2:615)	↑ Risk breast CA and malignant neoplasm of germ cell origin (Cancer Genet Cyogenet 1987;25:191)	Androgen supplementation to ↑ libido; surgical rx of gynecomastia
Turner's syndrome, gonadal dysgenesis	50% 45XO, 25% 45X/46XX; 25% have structurally abnormal X or Y or no detectable chromosomal abnormality (Am Rev Genet 1982;16:193)	Sexual infantilism, short stature, bilateral streak gonads, amenorrhea, webbed neck, shield chest, coarctation of aorta, lymphedema of hands and feet, epicanthal folds	↓ Estrogens and androgens, ↑ LH and FSH	If an XY cell line present, 30% risk of gonadal tumor (gonadoblastoma), 9% risk in others with Turner's syndrome.	Puberty can be induced by giving estrogen; growth hormone may accelerate short-term growth (Acta Pediatr Scand 1987;331(suppl):53); if Y cell line present, bilateral streak gonadectomy should be considered even in 45X

OTHER DISEASES IN CHILDREN

Table 13–1. (cont'd)

Disorder	Chromosomes	Presentation	Laboratory	Complications	Treatment
Mixed gonadal dysgenesis	45XO/46XY	Unilateral testis and contralateral streak gonad, persistent Müllerian structures, ambiguous genitalia, varying degrees of phallic enlargement, UG sinus, labioscrotal fusion, uterus, vagina, fallopian tube; 1/3–1/2 short in stature	↓ Testosterone, ↑ gonadotropins initially, testes secrete normal amounts of testosterone at puberty	↑ Risk gonadal and Wilms' tumors; 20% risk gonadoblastoma; Drash syn: sex ambiguity, Wilms' tumor, HT, proteinuria, progressive renal failure (J Pediatr 1976;585), infertile	2/3 raised as females, remove gonads, screen for Wilms' tumor, follow renal function
True hermaphrodite	2/3 46XX may be 46XX/46XY, 46XX/ 47XXYY, 46XY	Unilateral (40%) ovotestis on one side and ovary or testis on other, bilateral (20%) ovotestis on both sides, lateral (40%) testis on one side and ovary on other, ext genitalia masculinized to some extent, UG sinus		Hypospadias, labioscrotal fusion, clitoromegaly	2/3 raised as males, potential for fertility, following gender assignment, all contradictory gonads and internal duct structures removed

Condition	Karyotype	Clinical features	Labs	Risk	Treatment
Pure gonadal dysgenesis	46XX, 46XY	Phenotypic female of nl or tall stature with bilateral streak gonads, infantile internal and external genitalia, absent or retarded sexual maturation	↓ Estrogen	Those with XY gonadal dysgenesis at 30% risk of gonadoblastoma (Cancer 1986;57:1313)	Estrogen rx at expected time of puberty, remove gonads in XY
Bilateral vanishing testis syndrome	46XY	Absent or rudimentary testis, clinical appearance varies from complete female to that of male phenotype with microphallus and empty scrotum, if MIF produced prior to testicular loss no female internal structures	Castrate levels of testosterone, ↑ LH and FSH		Based on clinical appearance; phenotypic females treated with estrogen at puberty for secondary sex characteristics, may require vaginoplasty; phenotypic males treated with androgen replacement at puberty; possible testicular prosthesis
Male pseudohermaphrodite	46XY	Testes present, varying degrees of feminization phenotypically			

OTHER DISEASES IN CHILDREN

Table 13–1. (cont'd)

Disorder	Chromosomes	Presentation	Laboratory	Complications	Treatment
a. Disordered androgen synthesis	Defect in 1 of 5 enzymes needed for conversion of cholesterol to testosterone: 20,22 desmolase, 3BOH steroid dehydrogenase, 17 hydroxylase, 17,20 desmolase, 17 betahydroxysteroid dehydrogenase	If 17,20 desmolase or 17BOH steroid dehydrogenase usually phenotypic female, if less severe, male phenotype	↓ Testosterone and cortisol if 20,22 desmolase, 3BOH or 17 hydroxylase def; ↑ LH and FSH		Typically rear as per phenotypic appearance
b. 5-alpha-reductase	46XY	Normal male wolffian structures, female development of UG sinus and external genitalia; enlarged clitoris, UG sinus with separate vaginal and urethral openings and labioscrotal fusion; blind-ending short vagina, testes and epididymis located in labia, inguinal canal or abd, vas ends in the blind-ending vaginal pouch	Nl testosterone before and after HCG stimulation, deficient DHT response leading to markedly ↑ T/DHT response, cx of fibroblasts from genital skin demonstrates 5-alpha-reductase deficiency; ↑ testosterone at puberty		Depends on phenotypic findings and gender at time of dx, most raised as females, therefore need to remove gonads, estrogens at puberty, vaginoplasty, clitoral reduction; if male phenotypically at birth will partially masculinize at puberty,? if supraphysiologic estrogen levels help with phallic size, erectile functions (JCI 1984;74:1496)

c. Abnormal androgen receptor	46XY Deficient or defective androgen intracellular androgen receptor (protein). Also incl post-receptor defect of androgen resistance	Testicular feminization: Complete androgen insensitivity, nl female phenotype with ↓ axillary and pubic hair, internal genitalia absent, often present at puberty with amenorrhea, will feminize at puberty; Reifenstein synd: partial androgen insensitivity, penoscrotal hypospadias, UDTs, rudimentary wolffian duct derivs, gynecomastia, infertility. Rare, phenotypic nl infertile male	Nl serum testosterone, ↑ gonadotropins, ↑ estradiol	Infertility	Base on degree of genital ambiguity; testic female: delayed gonadectomy after puberty unless presence of palpable testes or testes associated with hernia
Persistent Müllerian duct syndrome, hernia uteri inguinale	46XY, defect in production of Müllerian-inhibiting substance	Nl-appearing male with female internal genitalia, bilateral fallopian tubes, uterus, upper vagina draining into prostatic utricle			Orchidopexy if necessary, preserving internal structures given their close proximity to vas (J Urol 1976;115:459)

OTHER DISEASES IN CHILDREN

Table 13–1. (cont'd)

Disorder	Chromosomes	Presentation	Laboratory	Complications	Treatment
Female pseudohermaphrodyte	46XX 3 etiol: (1) CAH, (2) maternal ingestion of androgens or androgen precursors, (3) maternal virilizing tumors	Virilization of external genitalia by abnl endocrine stimulation, varies from clitoral hypertrophy to nl-appearing penis and scrotum with palpable gonads; CAH: 3 enzymes responsible: (1) 11B hydroxylase defic: water retention, HT; (2) 21 hydroxylase defic: most common; if affects zona fasciculata and glomerulosa, most severe—hyponatremia, dehydration, acidosis, vascular collapse; (3) 3BOH steroid dehydrogenase defic: hyponatremia, dehydration	21 hydroxylase def: mild, increased 17OH progesterone, androstenedione and testosterone; severe, decreased cortisol and aldosterone, increased renin, 17OH progesterone, androstenedione and testosterone. 11B-hydroxylase: Increase deoxycorticosterone 3BOH steroid dehydrogenase; decreased aldosterone, cortisol, increased testosterone and androstenedione	High mortality with 3BOH steroid dehydrogenase	Surgical correction of virilized external genitalia

Crs: Usually identified at puberty in girls with amenorrhea. Ovarian function nl and fallopian tubes present (J Clin Endocrinol Metab 1973;36:634)

Cmplc: Infertility and sexual dysfunction. Surgical cmplc include need for regular dilation at home to prevent vaginal narrowing, inadequate vaginal length, vaginal stenosis, and dyspareunia (Int Surg 1987;72:45–47). When bowel segments are used, mucous drainage may be of concern

DiffDx: Imperforate hymen

Lab: As dictated by assoc abnl

Xray: Pelvic US indicated to assess uterus, ovaries, proximal vagina

Rx: Vaginoplasty. Timing variable. Some perform vaginoplasty in teenage years and others during early childhood (J Urol 1994;152:190). Vagina may be created from full-thickness skin flaps or by using isolated segment of ileum, sigmoid colon, or cecum (J Urol 1992;148:677)

Index

Prostatitis, 107–109
  and bacterial cystitis, 49
  NIH classification of, 107
Proteus mirabilis, in XGP, 15
Prune belly syndrome, 158–159
  vs. posterior urethral valves, 168
  and cryptorchidism, 180
  and vesicoureteral reflux, 147
PSA values, 115
Pseudosarcoma, *vs*. bladder cancer, 62
Psoriasis
  vs. balanoposthitis, 119
  vs. Reiter's syndrome, 74
Pure gonadal dysgenesis, intersex, *191*
Pyelonephritis
  acute, 10–12
  and bacterial cystitis, 49
  emphysematous, 12–13
  vs. malacoplakia, 17
  vs. renal abscess, 13
Pyelonephritis, xanthogranulomatous
    (XGP), 15–16

R
Rectocele, *vs*. cystocele, 68
Reinke crystals, and Leydig cell tumor,
    94
Reiter's syndrome, 74
  and gonorrhea, 75
Renal abscess, 13–14
Renal adenoma, 23–24
  vs. renal cell carcinoma, 29
Renal agenesis, 141–142
Renal angiomyolipoma, 25
Renal artery stenosis, *vs*.
    juxtaglomerular cell tumors, 26
Renal calculi, 34–36
Renal cell carcinoma (RCC), 28–30
  and acquired renal cystic disease, 46
  and xanthogranulomatous
    pyelonephritis, 16
  Robson staging system, 29
  vs. juxtaglomerular cell tumors, 26
  vs. renal adenoma, 23

vs. renal cyst, 42
vs. renal oncocytoma, 24
vs. renal sarcomas, 31
Renal cyst, 42–43
  Bosniak classification of, 42
  vs. juxtaglomerular cell tumors, 26
  vs. renal cell carcinoma, 29
Renal failure
  in acute pyelonephritis, 11
  in tuberculosis, 14
Renal insufficiency, and
    pheochromocytoma, 8
Renal lipoma, 26
Renal oncocytoma, 24
Renal pelvic tumors, 32–33
Renal sarcomas, 30–31
Renal scarring, in acute pyelonephritis,
    11
Renal trauma, 39–40
Renal tuberculosis, 14–15
Renal tubular acidosis, and
    urolithiasis, 34
Renal tumors. *See also* Renal cell
    carcinoma (RCC)
  juxtaglomerular, 26
  secondary, 31
  vs. renal abscess, 13
  vs. renal angiomyolipoma, 25
  vs. renal oncocytoma, 24
  vs. renal sarcomas, 31
Renal vein thrombosis, *vs*. autosomal
    recessive polycystic kidney
    disease, 45
Renin
  and juxtaglomerular cell tumor,
    26–27
  and renovascular hypertension,
    47
Renovascular hypertension, 47
Retrocaval ureter, 41
Retroperitoneal fibrosis, 22–23
Rhabdomyosarcoma, 183–184
  staging of, 183
Robson staging system, 29